"Thanks to Kino McGregor for this gift that makes yo_ _____ ___ ___ ___
ple regardless of age, gender, body type, or cultural or religious tradition. We
learn how to practice whether circumstances allow five minutes or five hours;
whether we are healthy, sick, injured, or even getting older. We are taught to
start where we are with what is here in the present and to work patiently and
slowly in order to grow the real lovingkindness of yoga—as we watch all of
our thoughts and ego stories in their continual relationship to our internal
breath and posture. Even from a modest beginning, learning to be so honestly
embodied reveals the profound relief, joy, and occasional fun that yoga is."

—Richard Freeman and Mary Taylor, authors of *The Art of Vinyasa*

"The representation and modifications in this book make my heart sing! A
must-have for all yoga practitioners!"

—Jessamyn Stanley, author of *Every Body Yoga*

"If you're looking to design a practice unique to your needs, lifestyle, and body,
then this is a great resource to begin! Filled with insightful information and
practical instructions, this is a book that meets people where they're at and
allows them to flourish. As someone who has advocated for yoga for *every*
body and everyone for over a decade, I'm thrilled to see this message growing
in power and scope. The more people who can get on the mat, the better!"

—Melanie Klein, editor of *Yoga Rising*

"This book represents a turning point in the history of yoga, and I'm moved
beyond words to see the whole of humanity represented here. What a gift Kino
is giving us by showing that yoga truly is for anyone who is interested in the
transformation and peace that yoga offers us all."

—Jivana Heyman, author of *Accessible Yoga*

"*Get Your Yoga On* is an accessible, diverse, and well-versed book that illustrates
the power of asana practice on our bodies, minds, and spirits. Kino's deep
knowledge of yoga, paired with her unique ability to make it approachable, are
beautifully displayed in this book and remind us that yoga is for every body."

—Sahara Rose Ketabi, best-selling author of *Eat Feel Fresh* and podcast host

• • • • • • ◆ • • • • • •

ALSO BY KINO MacGREGOR

GET YOUR YOUR YOGA ON

30 DAYS TO BUILD A PRACTICE
THAT FITS YOUR BODY AND YOUR LIFE

•••••••◆•••••••

KINO MacGREGOR

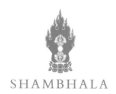

SHAMBHALA

Shambhala Publications, Inc.
4720 Walnut Street
Boulder, Colorado 80301
www.shambhala.com

Cover photos: Agathe Padovani
Cover design: Allison Meierding
Interior design: Allison Meierding

9 8 7 6 5 4 3 2 1

First Edition
Printed in the United States of America

♾ This edition is printed on acid-free paper that meets the
American National Standards Institute Z39.48 Standard.
♻ Shambhala Publications makes every effort to print on recycled paper.
For more information please visit www.shambhala.com.
Shambhala Publications is distributed worldwide by
Penguin Random House, Inc., and its subsidiaries.

Library of Congress Cataloging-in-Publication Data

Names: MacGregor, Kino, author.
Title: Get your yoga on: 30 days to build a practice that fits your body
and your life/Kino MacGregor.
Description: First edition. | Boulder, Colorado: Shambhala, 2020.
Identifiers: LCCN 2019045672 | ISBN 9781611807219 (trade paperback)
Subjects: LCSH: Hatha yoga. | Meditation. | Mind and body.
Classification: LCC RA781.7.M334 2020 | DDC 613.7/046—dc23
LC record available at https://lccn.loc.gov/2019045672

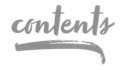

contents

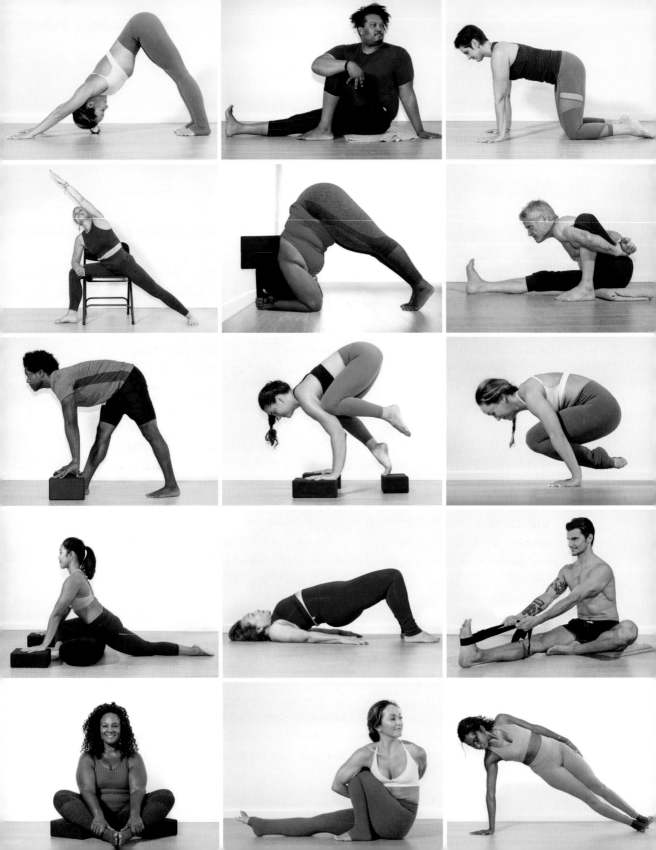

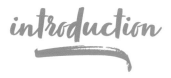

introduction

This is not another self-help book about manifesting your dreams with positive thinking; there are enough of those out there already. This is something else entirely. I am not here to tell you that everything you want will come true or that love always wins. It doesn't. Some dreams will never come true, some relationships just won't work out, some jobs you will not get, some things you cannot afford to buy. I am not here to talk to you about the miracles that will happen if only you believe in yourself fully. You, your life, and the world are infinitely more complex than that. Instead, I am here to offer you a path of true peace.

Yoga is such a widespread phenomenon that by now, nearly everyone has heard of it or tried it. Social media has spread the aspirational images of yogis to the farthest reaches of the world. Countless people of all ages have tried to stand on their heads, bend their backs, and twist their bodies because of what they've seen online. But many more have not, because they—like you and me—may doubt whether they have what it takes to be a yogi. Or you may have tried the poses and realized just how challenging they really are and were left feeling unworthy or excluded. Or you may be an avid practitioner looking to deepen and develop your practice but find the imagery of yoga shallow and superficial.

WELCOME TO YOUR YOGA PRACTICE!

This book relies on the power of this ancient practice to effect real change in your life. But that promise relies on you, not me. You have to practice. You have to put in the work. And perhaps more than anything else, you need to be a sincere seeker of the spiritual path. More than wanting to achieve your dreams, lose weight, make more money, find your perfect life partner, or reach any other material goal, to be a yoga practitioner you have to desire something much deeper. You must be so exhausted with chasing material success and measuring yourself by the standards of "the world" that you are willing to finally, at long last, turn your attention inward. You must burn with a desire for the ultimate, transcendent truth—truth beyond social identity, economic status, physical ableism, or any other standard based in this realm of mind and matter.

I've designed this book as a comprehensive and accessible yoga program based in the foundations of traditional yoga. This is a practice that is truly inclusive for all. Inspired by the popular yoga challenges that I host on Instagram, this book is an invitation to everyone to develop a personal yoga practice. The yoga challenge is so popular now that it can be considered more than a passing trend—it's a global movement. In 2019, "yoga challenge" was even ranked first on Google for fitness searches!

Yoga is for everyone. You don't need to be a young flexible dancer or a sleek athlete to do yoga. You also don't need a watered-down version of the practice to make it more palatable. You just need to be yourself and commit to practicing the thirty poses outlined in this book for at least five minutes a day for the rest of your life. Which ones you choose to practice on any given day is up to you—as long as you do at least five minutes of practice. Yoga challenge is a movement of real people who have directly experienced the benefits of the practice. You might not have the chance to give up everything and go to India to study with the masters or join an ashram, but I believe that you can carve out five minutes a day to practice. If you give the practice this small bit of time, you will lay the foundation for a whole new life.

WHY FIVE MINUTES?

Why five minutes? Well, five minutes is the minimum amount of time that you need to reset the habitual patterns of the body and mind. It's also a measurement of time that even the busiest person can fit into their day. You can definitely practice more than that. But so many people think they have to give two hours to a sweaty full-on practice or it's not worth practicing at all. I know many yogis and fitness enthusiasts who stop practicing when their life situation changes due to work or family; they just didn't have the time to commit to a lengthy practice. Or new students to yoga can often feel overwhelmed by the idea of doing yoga continuously for an hour or more. It feels like a marathon, and it may not fit into your life. But everyone can squeeze five minutes into their schedule.

Studies show tangible health benefits to exercising for just five minutes a day. A study published by the American College of Cardiology examined more than fifty-five thousand adults, looking at exercise habits over fifteen years, and found that people who were even slightly active had much stronger hearts and lungs and lived up to three years longer as compared to those who didn't exercise at all.* Even modest physical exertion can improve your mood and help you sleep at night.

Yoga is more than just physical fitness. It is a spiritual path of inner transformation that works slowly, over many years, to change the operating system of your brain. Not only does the practice teach you to calm your nervous system in the moment of practice but also how to apply the same tools amid difficult life situations. Instead of operating from the fear-based mentality that assumes the world is a big competition for a limited few slots at the top of the heap, you learn how to be at peace with yourself wherever you are in the grand scope of life. Much like getting a new operating system changes everything about your computer, yoga practice—even for as little as five minutes a day—installs a new operating system in your brain that gives you a whole new paradigm.

Finally, if you want you to change your behavior, start with a daily ritual. Behavior that is ritualized takes less mental energy to do every day. It becomes a part of who you are, like brushing your teeth.

A THIRTY-POSE JOURNEY

Rather than giving you any time frame to complete this yoga challenge, I designed this book as a complete practice and journey into some key yoga poses. You could speed through the poses and string them all together to create one flow. Or you could spend weeks, months, or years on each pose. Or you could do both!

If you're just starting the practice, I advise you to follow the poses in the order laid out and not skip ahead to one of the poses that looks more interesting or easy. I ask you to stay in moments of difficulty and face the challenge of each pose with kindness, love, and perseverance. While you may be tempted to give yourself a pass or fail grade on each pose, that is not the purpose of this challenge. Instead, I encourage you to focus on the learning available within each pose.

A CHALLENGE, NOT A COMPETITION

While this book presents a yoga challenge, I do not want you to take the word *challenge* too literally. Yoga practice is not a zero-sum game with winners and losers. There is not a scarcity of asanas or spiritual evolution. There is no timeline

---

* Lee, Duck-chul et al., "Leisure-Time Running Reduces All-Cause and Cardiovascular Mortality Risk," *Journal of the American College of Cardiology* 64, no. 5 (August 2014): doi: 10.1016/j.jacc.2014.04.058.

to beat, prize for finishing first, or punishment for finishing last. There is, perhaps, no finishing. So much cultural conditioning demands us to run at full speed toward external achievement. Many of us, including myself, feel so much pressure to fit into societal standards for beauty, happiness, and success, and we feel stuck despite massive effort. It may seem odd to hear this statement coming from someone who has been dedicated to yoga for over twenty years. I've been driven to meet some pretty high external metrics (many of which I haven't met). These "goals" hang over my head and either motivate me to keep going (on good days) or tell me I'm not good enough (on bad days).

Now, I know it isn't true. I'm sharing this so you can see how ridiculous the paradigm of worldly achievement is. It's never enough. No one is ever good enough, and there is always another hurdle to jump over. We are obsessed with being the best, and we think achievement will make us happy. We achieve success by many factors: belief, privilege, luck, hard work, perseverance, timing, grace. But success measured by worldly standards is temporary.

As we begin the journey of yoga together, I encourage you to shift your paradigm. Choose love. Choose presence. Choose beingness. In a world that defines your worth by what you do and how you do it, the decision to love unconditionally is a revolution. Love is a choice, but it's also innate, inherent, and indestructible. People say love is blind. I don't think it is. I think love sees clearly and perfectly and accepts it all. So, I hope you will take this yoga challenge together with me from a totally new perspective. This isn't a race. In fact, in this yoga challenge, I invite you to drop out of the race to be number one and choose to love yourself exactly as you are.

A PRACTICE FOR ALL OF US

Sometimes yoga asanas can seem a little daunting, but yoga is for all of us. We are flooded with images of young, flexible, slim bodies doing poses that seem gravity defying and quite frankly impossible. These images make yoga practice seem like an exclusive club of which only the very fit, very young, and very flexible can be a part.

It is important to remember that yoga is a combination of a great many things, including breath, focus, meditation, self-study, asanas, and ultimately connection. Yoga is the art and science of getting to know yourself. Yet, while yoga is a practice that can be done by anyone, some forms of asanas can be exclusionary. Every body functions differently. Some of us come to the physical practice with injuries and limitations, but that should not exclude us from asana practice. Your body—which you may have often looked at with judgment or hatred and wished was something else—is your best friend, your door to liberation, and your pathway to peace.

Throughout this book you will find modifications that aim to make all the poses accessible for every body. Not only will you see different variations of the poses themselves but also different students demonstrating the poses. Representation matters, and it has been a conscious effort on my part to include a true diversity of size, shape, age, and ethnicity. Inclusivity cannot be a mere statement; action must follow. For the first time in any of my books you will see me only occasionally. Instead, the focus will be on the beautiful students whose practice I hope you will be inspired by. I hope you see yourself reflected back in these pages and be motivated to practice. Accessibility and inclusivity unlock yoga's true potential to change the world, and that starts with you!

In yoga we need to see someone who looks like us doing asanas to believe that we can do it too. When I first started practicing, all the high-level teachers featured in videos and workshops were tall guys with long limbs and big muscles. When I saw them lift up, I didn't believe that I could do it too. No one doing lift-ups or teaching looked like me. In fact, I had people tell me my thighs were too big and my arms too small to ever hope at getting into some of the poses. I had to decide to focus on the tiny voice of faith inside me instead of the very loud voice of doubt.

• • • • • • ◆ • • • • • •

The deepest, truest yoga that I know is internal and can't ever be judged from the outside. We *all* have our limitations and obstacles. The journey is about how we face those struggles and what love we cultivate in our hearts along the way. My hope for you in this yoga challenge is that you truly get established in a lifelong spiritual journey.

May this practice bring peace, joy, and love into your life. When you begin to experience the flow of positive energy that yoga brings, you will be bubbling over with happiness. May each practice session bring you deeper into alignment with all the goodness in the world. May your heart be open and filled with compassion. May your mind be clear and filled with wisdom. May you be blessed with grace and may your light grow brighter with each breath. May you practice yoga and change your world, one breath at a time.

GET
YOUR
YOGA
ON

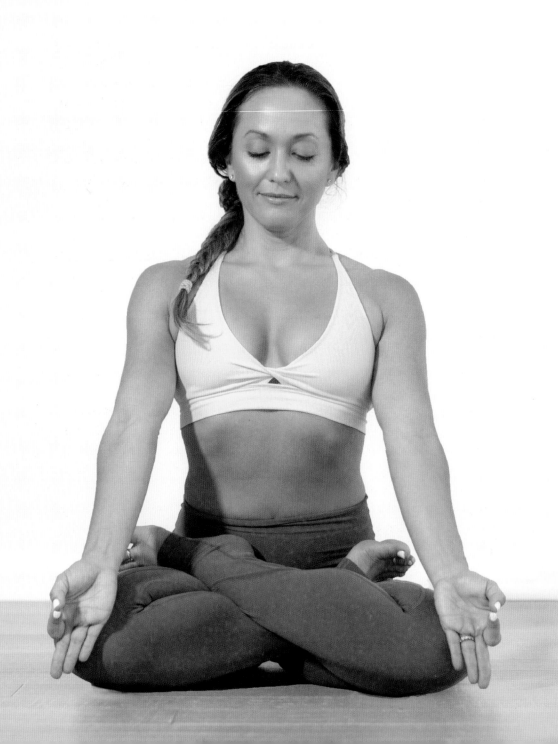

The Origins of Yoga

....

Contemporary Western yoga practice may not make this obvious, but yoga is an ancient science of the soul with roots deep in India's history. While there is much debate about what yoga looked like thousands of years ago, one thing is certain: the intention of all ancient practices of yoga was rooted in a desire to know the deepest truth about one's own life, God, and the universe. Yoga is deeply tied to Hinduism, yet yoga today is often portrayed as far from its source. In a time when the popularity of yoga is rising and the imagery around yoga speaks more to mainstream Western culture, it is absolutely necessary that we learn about the essential nature of this potent practice.

Yoga in Sanskrit literally translates to *yuj*, or to "yoke," and is commonly interpreted as meaning unity. But traditionally, unity is both a source of liberation and bondage. For example, in Patanjali's Yoga Sutras, uniting or conflating the material with the spiritual is noted as the source of suffering, whereas experiencing unity of the spirit (*purusha*) with the spirit of God (*Ishvara purusha*) is considered the foundation of liberation. So, unity is not enough. A yogi must be conscious of what the mind is united with and seek to place it in unity with the highest source of knowledge—the all-pervading light of God.

There is ample evidence from traditional Hindu texts regarding the spiritual origin and intention of yoga. The *Hatha Yoga Pradipika*, dating from 1500 C.E., is an in-depth study of asanas, pranayama, mudra, and samadhi, and the first text to present yoga asanas in a concrete form. It couches the physical practice within the framework of *hatha*, which literally translates as "sun and moon." And it defines the goal of yoga as the development of subtle energy and samadhi, or the experience of deep meditative absorption.

Yoga is distinguished within the six main schools of orthodox Indian thought by its foundation and emphasis on personal practice. The thread of these philosophical schools is united around what is called the *sanatana dharma*, or the "eternal truth." While in the past yoga was practiced primarily by men of the Brahmin caste, it is an equal opportunity path with the sole requirement of consistent and dedicated practice. As such, it is this foundational principle that allows anyone, regardless of race, religion, sexual orientation, or gender, to achieve *moksha*, the liberation that is the essence of yoga. Each person is charged with personal responsibility for their actions along the path of yoga, and their progress is defined by their own actions, words, and thoughts.

According to Patanjali's Yoga Sutras 1.14, a firm foundation in yoga is defined by three things:

1. Commitment to the practice over a long time with many years of unwavering dedication (*dirga kala*).
2. Continuity of practice on and off the mat. Not only must you do the asanas regularly but you must also translate the lessons learned on your mat to your life (*nairantarya*).
3. Intention in your practice. You have to yearn for the spiritual realization and be a sincere seeker (*satkara*).

Starting during British colonial rule, the practice of yoga in India was banned and yogis were portrayed in a negative light. Yogis were seen as rebels who challenged the puritanical paradigm of Victorian society. The British Raj used the word *fakir* to refer to yogis in a derogatory manner, despite the word's association with Muslim mystics. This reference solidified yogis as outcasts from society. After the British colonial period ended, yoga's resurgence was led by a few lineage-based Indian teachers who found an audience in Western yoga students. These teachers, including Sri Tirumalai Krishnamacharya, B. K. S. Iyengar, and K. Pattabhi Jois, among others, paved the way for yoga to slowly make its way into the Western world. Now, years later, we are at a critical turning point for the world of yoga.

As Western students of yoga, we have a choice. We can continue to practice the poses and let the journey stop there. We can allow ourselves to be complicit in a system of cultural appropriation where the profits of the ancient tradition of yoga fall primarily into American or European multinational corporations. Or we can use the tool of yoga as a catalyst for a true revolution by letting yoga be a clarion call to create a better, more just, and equitable world. My hope in sharing this yoga challenge with you is to help you access the rich cultural history of yoga, and to invite you to join me not only in the practice of asanas but also the transformative, revolutionary view that the yoga path offers.

Let's Get Started!

Some people think that the purpose of yoga is to feel good. While it's true that when you practice yoga long term you will experience a deep and lasting peace, you do not arrive on your mat to feel good per se. Instead, yoga asks you first to feel. Just feel. Whether pain or pleasure, happiness or sadness, you are here to feel it all. Yoga is about what you learn on the mat and how you apply those lessons to change your world.

Feeling the physical body is often the beginning of an awakening of consciousness sparked by yoga. But the physical is only the beginning. The mind has the potential to feel much more than just what the nerves register as sensation. Sensations themselves range from gross, solidified, and dense to undulating, shimmering, and more rarefied. Muscles, bones, joints, and the whole network of physicality can be felt and experienced as a world of wonder if you allow your mind to dive in through the door of yoga. Thoughts and emotions have a kind of vibration that can be felt as an extra-sensory perception resonating within the body. After the mind is able to perceive physical sensations, thought, and emotions, there is an even deeper level that borders on the mystical. I often refer to this experience as the *inner body*, or the body of energy and light.

Before you write this concept off as hippie woo-woo magic and file it away next to unicorns and elves, think about this—contemporary physics has discovered that matter is, at its most basic and indivisible level, comprised primarily of empty space. At the subatomic level, where electrons zip around the protons and neutrons in the nucleus, the majority of what exists is nothing. Pause and take that in for a moment. Your body, this book, and every single material object is made of *emptiness*. The fundamental quality that defines all things is not really there at all. Ancient yogis described the feeling of directly sensing the smallest most indivisible particle of matter, which they called the *anu*. One can only assume that their minds were able to feel, perceive, and experience the space between the subatomic particles that is the reality of the innermost body. You too, with years of practice, will be able to feel the pulsating, vibrating, radiating sensations that can only arise when you truly descend into the inner body. Here, in the mystical space of the world within, you possess a microscope so powerful there is nothing it cannot see. Some people have questioned whether the presence of God can be felt in the vast empty space. If you are a spiritual seeker, then perhaps you will use the tool of yoga to answer that question for yourself.

This book is offering you a yoga challenge—a road map to a spiritual path that will challenge you to work with your mind and intention, befriend your body, use your breath and heart mindfully, and bring your unique light into the world.

Like any worthwhile journey, you can expect to go through highs and lows. There will be days when you feel as though you don't want to practice anymore. Other days, you will feel tired and sore. Trust that it's all part of the process. You are here to grow spiritually, to expand your heart, and to heal. Along the way there are inevitable ups and downs. It's important that you take these as signs of growth, not failure. In fact, you can never fail at yoga! All you need to succeed is to keep practicing.

Here I will explain the important points for you to keep in mind and heart as you take on this yoga challenge.

ASANAS ARE TOOLS

Yoga poses confront you. You meet your tightness, weakness, and all other sorts of limitations on the mat. And between your breath and your body, there is no escape. This self-inquiry is a vital part of the learning process of yoga.

When I first started practicing, I thought that the more advanced the asana, the more spiritual learning it held. It's easy to think like that when you first start. The yoga poses are what often attract people to the practice, but they are tools, not goals or ends in and of themselves. If you focus too much on the poses, you risk creating a kind of rat-race mentality where you try to collect more and more poses in order to be a "better" yogi. Equating spiritual development with physical proficiency can set up a hierarchy of extreme ableism that undermines the healing potential of yoga. It took me many years of practice to see through that illusion.

Some poses are not better just because they appear to be more rigorous or difficult. It's not about how far you can push but rather developing a deep intelligence in the body that feels, sees, hears, and loves every fiber of your being. In Cobra Pose (*Bhujangasana*), for example, it may seem like not a lot is going on. But if you dive into the sensation of your inner body, you might feel each joint of your spine lifting and creating space; your pelvic floor awakening like a fire; the muscles of your middle and upper back beginning to fold like a caterpillar; and perhaps even a rising sensation like a waterfall along your spinal axis. Likewise, the healing journey of backbends begins with your intention to dive into the depths of your being. Sometimes that means following the expression to some place physically deep, but sometimes not. For me, practice is devotion, dedication, and depth, a quiet place I return to worship every day. There are days when it's not fun, but those days can often be profound and healing.

PAY ATTENTION TO YOUR BREATH

It took me years before I understood just how important the breath is to yoga practice. Some people can perform quite exciting asanas but they are unable to breathe deeply. Similarly, other students may not perform asanas deeply but their breath demonstrates a penetrating inner focus. While it may be tempting to associate proficiency in asanas with deep yoga, the truth of the matter is that yoga practice is an inner experience. While we can never measure or judge someone's spirituality from the outside, the breath gives us a window to peer into the often-obscured realm of the spirit.

The breath is the thread that ties the conscious and subconscious together. By tuning in to your breath, you have a window into the deepest layers of your mind. Even more, the mysteries of life and death are contained within inhalation and exhalation. The faculty of the breath is the power that illuminates the body with the vibrance of life. Without the breath, there is quite simply no life.

An old yogi myth states that each individual's life span is defined by the total amount of breaths allotted to them on this journey. When those breaths are finished, the journey ends. If you have had the grace to be present when a soul is born into a human body, you've seen the miracle of the breath bring life to the body. Similarly, if you have been present when a being breathes their last breath out and life leaves the body, you've witnessed another miracle. The breath is life, and intimacy with the breath brings wisdom and attunement to the rarefied realm of the spirit.

Chale vate chalam chittam nishchale nishchalam bhavet yogi sthanutvamapnoti tato vayum nirodhayet.

When the breath moves, *chitta*, the mental force, also moves. When the breath is still, chitta is also still. By stabilizing and controlling the breath, the yogi stabilizes and controls the mind.

—*HATHA YOGA PRADIPIKA 2.2*

My teacher said that the entire purpose of the asanas is to create a field of experience for you to breathe. The breath is the magic catalyst for the inner world. Without a deep full breath, the asanas are just body bending. Use each pose as an opportunity to breathe deeply. Let the shape of the pose be a secondary experience to the depth of your breath. During asana practice, the breath resonates, creating deep breathing with sound. The audible breath allows you to hear and feel your breath more powerfully. It also allows your breath to resonate within the emptiness of your inner body.

The breath in yoga—*prana vayu* in Sanskrit—is more closely related to the winds of our life force than simply taking in oxygen. There is a type of breath associated with every emotional state. Anger and anxiety are often associated with short, shallow, rapid breaths. Sadness, depression, and hopelessness are characterized by long exhalations or sighs. Happiness, joy, and love are shown by deep, rhythmic diaphragmatic breaths. During your practice you will notice that certain poses trigger different types of breathing. Proficiency in asanas is demonstrated as much by the ability to breathe deeply as it is by the ability to bend the body. Place your emphasis on the inner experience of the breath and there will be no limit to how deeply your practice will go.

PRANA VAYU PRACTICE

The breathing technique for traditional yoga that I share with you here is relatively simple, yet infinitely complex. Draw your lower belly in toward your spine and activate your pelvic floor. Keep your lips sealed. Place the tip of your tongue on the roof of your mouth behind your two front teeth. Relax the back of your throat and your soft palette. Engage your vocal chords slightly. Breathing through your nose, say "Sa" as you inhale and "Ha" as you exhale. You might find that you sound like Darth Vader, but don't worry, I promise you won't go over to the dark side. Keep your lower belly drawn in and breathe from your diaphragm. It may feel like your breath is traveling through a straw placed at the center of your spine.

Equalize the length of each breath, so that if you breathe in for five seconds, you also breath out for five seconds. During asana practice it is not advisable to breathe in for longer than ten seconds or less than one second.

Within that range you are welcome to find a breath pattern that works for you in each asana. During your practice each day, I encourage you to place careful emphasis on the depth and quality of your breath. Start off each practice with at least five deep breaths before you begin to attempt any of the asanas. Let your breath be the beginning of your practice. The spark of your breath helps ignite the inner fire of purification and awareness. Then, as the awareness of your breath becomes more natural, try to be aware of your breath in all moments of your life. Notice when your breath changes from moment to moment, depending on various life situations. Let this be a route into your inner world.

PRACTICE MINDFULLY

Start your spiritual journey from a paradigm of wholeness. You come to the practice to experience the truth of your inner being. There is no need to rush or judge yourself harshly along the way. Understand that it never matters how well you do a pose; the quality of your effort is most important. Cultivate an attitude of mindfulness and learn to be aware of all the sensations of your body. Your goal is to feel everything without any judgment. You may be drawn to spend more time in silent, quiet reflection. As you practice, place an emphasis on objectivity and simply allow your sensations to be what they are without judging them. It is easy to label things as good or bad; it's harder to allow things to be just what they are. This is the practice of mindfulness. Pure observation—free from the story you are drawn to tell about why things are the way they are, and whether they are good or bad—sets you free to truly be present with your body, your mind, and ultimately with the whole world.

When practicing the yoga poses, you will be tempted to judge yourself by how well you can perform the shapes. But I think by now you can really see that this performative mind-set is not yoga's essence or promise. The poses are merely vehicles for experience. As you flow the poses outlined here, cultivate an attitude of mindful presence and call yourself into a greater, more whole sense of embodiment. Let the felt sense of your body exactly as it is be enough. Try it in any pose and you will lay the foundations of peace deep within your heart. You can practice mindfulness in any situation in your life as well. The paradigm of the equanimous mind will decrease your reactivity and perhaps lead to new insights, increased productivity, and more happiness.

LOVING-KINDNESS MEDITATION

Yoga practice naturally opens your heart. You may feel that this tender aching vulnerability is strange and new. In order to get more acquainted with the power of an open heart, I suggest that at the end of every practice, you sit quietly in a comfortable seated meditation pose and bring your attention to your heart-center. End each practice by carefully recalibrating your mind with the active practice of thinking new thoughts. Start off by sending love, peace, joy, and forgiveness to yourself. With each breath in, feel your heart. Then, with each breath out, say, "May I be peaceful." Let only one feeling be associated with one breath. Then extend your heart and send those same blessings to a friend or family member. Call up the image of a dear one for whom you feel natural love and concern. Then, in the same way, with each breath in, feel your heart. With each breath out say, "May you be peaceful." Next, extend the same feelings to all beings, human and nonhuman, all over the world and all through the universe. Open your heart to the vast expanse of all living beings. With each breath in, feel your heart. With each breath out say, "May all beings throughout time and space, including myself, be peaceful." Continue with the same group of phrases for each set of beings to whom you open your heart. Don't worry if it doesn't feel natural. Just like anything, it gets better with practice.

There is an advanced form of loving-kindness practice called *tonglen* that originates from the Tibetan Buddhist tradition. Tonglen is the practice of sending love to people with whom you have a grievance. Much as Jesus advised his disciples to love their enemies and pray for people who persecuted them, the practice of sending love to difficult people is an integral part of spiritual practice. In order to truly send love to all beings you have to be willing to send love to *all* people, even the ones whom you find challenging. This is a yoga challenge after all. When you feel strong enough and ready to let some of the old hurt go, call to mind your difficult person. Perhaps start with a simple version of the loving-kindness meditation that says, "May you come out of your misery." Continue with, "May you find the spiritual path, grow, and evolve from your current state." If you feel up for it, add in, "May I forgive you." Finally, end with, "May you be happy and peaceful." While it might seem counterintuitive to send good wishes to your enemies, I think we can all agree that miserable people make the world a more miserable place. If the person who was problematic to you truly found the happiness and peace of the spiritual path, the world would be a better place. We can all wish for that.

Once you establish the practice of loving-kindness meditation, you can do it anywhere. As you're on the way to that holiday gathering, practice generating loving-kindness toward yourself and all attendees. As you wait in long lines at department stores, generate loving-kindness toward yourself and all other shoppers and employees. In this way you will make the world a more loving, kinder place for yourself and those around you.

HONOR YOUR BODY

Sometimes I fall into the trap of equating a thin body with beauty. Do you? Well, if you do, you're not alone. No matter how many times you hear that myth debunked, it's hard not to fall right back into the trap. All you have to do is look at conventional images presented by media and brands and you can end up in a tailspin of negative body image.

I can't tell you how many women have told me that they were inspired by my strength because I'm not a tall, skinny person. Well, let me offer my muscular thighs and petite height as inspiration for all the other short, thick bodies out there. And let me tell all the tall, skinny people, you are beautiful too. (I married a tall, skinny person!) Whether you are young or old, the practice is for you. No matter what size, shape, ethnicity, religion, gender, political affiliation, nationality, socioeconomic class, yoga is for you. The only thing that you really need to do is get on your mat (or a beach towel, or a rug) for as little as five minutes a day.

The perfect body for yoga practice is the one you have. Learn to love it and celebrate it with every breath and you will find so much peace within yourself. So much of the real challenge of yoga is learning to love your body. Let this practice bring you into the freedom of truly experiencing the oneness of your body, mind, and soul. In a world that tells you you're not good enough, the decision to love yourself is a revolution. Be a revolutionary in your own mind. It's up to you to stand up for what you're worth. If you don't see it, feel it, and honor it, then the world outside of you won't either.

EAT MINDFULLY

You may be inspired to take a mindful look at your diet as you begin to practice yoga. As you begin to feel your body more, it's only natural that you want to nourish and heal your body. Food is an intimate communication between you and your body. If you feel inspired to make dietary shifts, be sure that your intention is rooted in love. Don't import the diet and weight loss culture to your yoga world. Instead, base your decisions on a desire to love your body and your world. When I first started practicing yoga over twenty years ago, I made the decision to follow a plant-based diet. You may be inspired to do something similar. But if not, that's OK too. I recommend all yoga practitioners simply bring as much conscious awareness into their dietary choices as possible and use the body as a laboratory for the success or failure of any diet.

As a yogi it's important to have an attitude of mindfulness around your food. Avoid eating while you're distracted by things such as streaming videos or TV. Avoid rushing through your meals while on the go. While you may not be able to sit down at a table and share a family-oriented meal, especially if you work multiple jobs, I encourage you to find time to bring presence into every aspect of your life, including mealtime. You don't need to climb to a remote mountaintop to appreciate your food as you eat. On a five-minute break amid a busy day, find a quiet spot, perhaps outside in a small patch of sun, if that is accessible, and let your mealtime be a moment of mindfulness. Then you'll return to work with even more presence. If your family is big and rowdy, see if you can share the practice of presence with them during a meal, and you might create even more connection between loved ones. Simply bring the same quality of awareness that you practice during yoga to your eating habits. There is no dogma or right method, so I encourage you to find what works for you.

MINDFUL EATING EXERCISE

As you sit down to eat, pause and reflect on everything that made your meal possible. Contemplate all the plants, animals, insects, humans, sunlight, air, water, and everything that brought the components of your meal into being. Then actively send a thank-you to each step in the process. Feel your heart saying "thank you" and bowing down to each and every being that made your food possible. Then, as you eat, chew slowly, breathe between bites of food. Let the taste explode in your mouth and appreciate each flavor. Make this exercise a prayer of love, gratitude, and appreciation.

LET YOUR LIFE REFLECT YOUR YOGA VALUES

Yoga is a path of awakening. It begins as a personal journey. You feel better when you start practicing because your heart opens. First that shows up as self-love, but it doesn't stop there. Enlightenment is often described by the spiritual teachers of India as an action taken for the benefit of all beings. The premise is that spiritual awakening is equal parts wisdom and compassion. Wisdom wakes you up, compassion compels you to share the light with others.

There are so many ways you can show up as a yogi and take a stand for a kinder, more peaceful and loving world. But you have to do the work of dedicated, devotional spiritual practice, or sadhana. You must commit yourself to the sometimes painful and rude process of waking yourself up out of the slumber of conditioned existence. You have to be willing to see all your darkness, all the places you have been complicit in injustice, all the ways you have intentionally or unintentionally caused harm to yourself and others. And you must work tirelessly to evolve beyond that. When your light grows brighter, you make the world a better place. But it doesn't stop there. Whatever awakening, whatever shift has happened in your heart becomes real when you take action that aligns with your newfound realizations. Without concrete action built around consequence, all the lofty ideas are just that, ideas. There is no spiritual bypass for bringing home the lessons of the yogi life. You have to be willing to work equally as hard in your life as you work in your practice.

Some people question me when I get fiery or take a stance on issues in the world. Well, I cannot really apologize for that. I'm taking the lessons of my practice off my mat and into my life. To me, compassionate thoughts backed up with enlightened action is what this practice is about. If you truly want to make the world a peaceful place, then do the work to make it so. Yoga is not a panacea for all your problems. But it certainly can be a catalyst for major life transformation. By clearing your mind, opening your heart, and loving your body, you are contributing to the evolution of the planet in a small but immensely meaningful way.

SHOW UP FOR PRACTICE EVERY DAY

Just because I've been practicing yoga for over twenty years doesn't mean that I wake up every day filled with enthusiasm to practice. I think about yoga as one of the foundational relationships of my life. I have a relationship with my practice, and just like any long-term committed relationship, I go through phases with it. When I first started practicing, I went through what you could call the "honeymoon" period of practice. During that time, I just couldn't get enough yoga. I would eat, breathe, and sleep yoga if I could. I tried to recruit every person I spoke with to come to class with me because yoga was just the best thing ever. After I finished practice, I would hang out with yoga friends and talk about yoga. Then when I went home, I would read books about yoga. I would even dream about yoga!

Since then, I've gone through cycles of doubt, disillusionment, boredom, laziness, and general neglect. I have also experienced deepening, maturing, ripening, subtlety, grace, peace, wisdom, and love. Through it all, the single defining feature of my life has been that I have managed to get on my yoga mat approximately six days a week for the last twenty years. The practice is the essence of what I've committed myself to, and I have not really wavered in that. Not every practice has been monumental. Most practices in fact have been humble and quiet. Some were certainly sloppy and lazy. Others still were gentle and modified. But it's all practice.

* * * * * * ◆ * * * * * *

You will want to quit. You will be sore. You will experience doubt. It's up to you to keep going. Just practice. Show up on your mat when you're tired, energized, happy, sad, whatever. Practice changes the way you think and feel, and because of that it literally changes your world. I personally think it's extraordinary enough to devote a little time each day to your practice because when you practice, you shine that much brighter.

Practice is not performance. Practice is just practice; a daily ritual of spiritual self-inquiry. Practice defines itself by the sheer power of repetition over many years—an inner journey that unfolds in pieces. It's not always something that lifts you up. Sometimes you want to quit, sometimes you feel emotions bubbling up, sometimes you are just sore. But still you practice. It's not perfection. Or rather, in all its many flaws and fumbles there is true perfection. Big changes are often experienced in small things. When you practice yoga and change your world, the transformation may show up in the details. Look for them and celebrate every step forward.

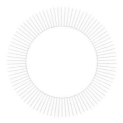

TUNE IN TO YOUR INTENTION

Yoga is . . .

A promise of peace.

A path of healing.

A journey to the center of yourself.

A discipline of truth and God realization.

A daily devotion, sadhana.

A prayer.

A physical practice with a spiritual intention.

An ancient science of the soul.

A ritual in service of the Divine.

A quiet space of worship.

A reclaiming of the sacred.

A life of inner peace.

An act of faith that chooses the spiritual and the unseen, over the material
  and the seen.

A training of mind to turn infinitely inward.

A rock to rest upon in times of chaos and hardship.

A decision to be stronger, to change the world, one breath at a time.

A moving meditation where the answers to life's most difficult questions
  are answered by the breath.

A path of love and forgiveness.

Yoga is all this and more. It's important that you finish the sentence with what yoga is to you. Each of us defines yoga for ourselves when we practice. It can be so easy to get sidetracked from the path and caught in a web of desire. Take time each day and remember what yoga is to you and why you practice.

◆◆◆◆◆◆ ◆ ◆◆◆◆◆◆

So, are you ready to begin? By practicing these poses and opening the door to the spiritual journey of yoga, your life will change. In the space between the breath and the body, in the quiet world of inner light, you will experience a peace that surpasses all understanding. Like a mythological hero, you will return forever changed, empowered by your experiences, imbued with a timeless wisdom. Remember, it doesn't matter how well you do the poses. It only matters that you try. The quality of your effort matters more than the results. Don't judge, don't quit. Just feel, just try. I believe in you, and I hope you are ready to believe in yourself.

The
Practice

Downward-Facing Dog

Adho Mukha Svanasana

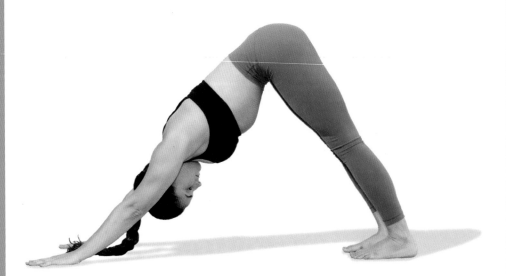

1

Downward-Facing Dog, represented in all styles of yoga, is one of the most universal and fundamental poses. When people picture yoga in their minds, they often think of Downward-Facing Dog. Known as *Adho Mukha Svanasana* in most yoga traditions, and sometimes just as *Chatuari* (Fourth Position) in the Ashtanga method, Downward-Facing Dog is one of the most beneficial and accessible poses. This asana forms the foundational key point in the Sun Salutations, a popular warm-up used in many styles of yoga and is often used as a "rest" in-between other asanas, such as *Chaturanga Dandasana*.

Some students, particularly advanced practitioners, may find Downward-Facing Dog to be quite easy, but the truth is that it can be a very challenging posture. Downward-Facing Dog can be difficult if you have tight shoulders, sore or arthritic wrists, and tight hamstrings. It can also be challenging if you lack the strength to hold yourself up in this position.

I have included at least one Downward-Facing Dog in every yoga practice I've done or taught for over twenty years. And this is where we begin our yoga challenge journey together as well.

Unroll your yoga mat or claim a space in your home to begin your practice today. Start off in a comfortable seated position. Close your eyes, tune in to your body by bringing your attention to the quiet space of listening at the center of your heart. Feel your breath moving in and out of your body. Then gently place your hands in prayer position, resting your thumbs at the center of your sternum. Allow a consciously deep inhalation to enter your lungs, then exhale as you resonate the sound OM. It could be as soft as a whisper or loud enough to fill the room; it depends on you. But let the sonic presence open your heart, clear your mind, and create a sacred space of worship and reverence. Bask in it for a few moments. Then slowly open your eyes.

Gently come on to your hands and knees, aligning your hands with your shoulders and your feet with your hips for Tabletop Pose, a common preparatory pose that you will return to repeatedly to set up for many yoga poses.

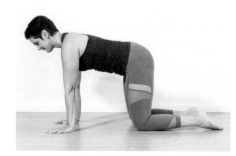

Curl your toes under and gently spread your fingers. Drawing in your lower belly and activating your pelvic floor, gently straighten your legs by sending your hips back and up. Pivot inside of your hip joints to rotate your pelvis back to the hint of an anterior tilt. Let your sitting bones lift slightly and ground your heels as much as possible. Roll your shoulder blades away from each other and down your back to give space to your neck. Activate your deltoids and latissimus dorsi muscles to stabilize your shoulders. Soften

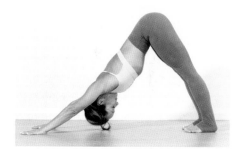

your neck and gaze gently toward your navel. Count out five long deep breaths. Keep your lower belly tucked in as you breathe.

Place your knees back on the ground, lower down to *Balasana* (Child's Pose) (see later in this chapter, page 21). Finally, roll all the way over onto your back, lie down, and close your eyes. Spread your legs and your arms, settle your sacrum on the floor, and relax into the Final Relaxation (sometimes called *Savasana*, or Corpse Pose) (see page 142). Feel your body weight releasing into the ground. Stay for at least one minute but up to ten minutes. When you feel rested and renewed, return to a comfortable seated position. Keeping your eyes closed and your mind attuned to your inner body, end with a long, deep conscious breath in and exhale the holy vibration OM.

VARIATIONS
Downward-Facing Dog for Bigger Bodies

This variation of Downward-Facing Dog is very close to the traditional representation you often see in mainstream yoga culture. In order to make this pose more accessible for a larger body, take a larger stance to distribute the weight more evenly. One of the first steps in creating asana variations for larger bodies is to go bigger in the asana, which offers more room for the body.

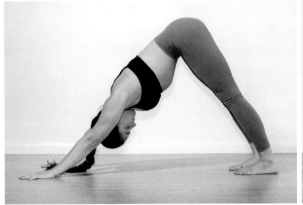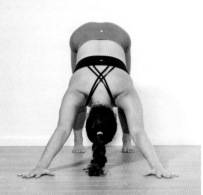

From Tabletop Pose, take your hands much wider; bring your pinkie fingers right to the edge of your mat. Your outer shoulders will line up with the center of your wrists, which may even place your ring fingers and pinkies off the mat. Line the creases of your wrists up with the top edge of your mat. Root down through the knuckles of your hands. Take your knees as wide as your mat. Curl your toes under, firm your abs by squeezing your belly and lift your hips up and back. You are now in the shape of a big inverted V.

Bend your elbows, rotate your upper arms, engage your triceps, and gently push the floor away from you. Root down through your legs. Your heels don't need to touch the floor as long as you are feeling a sense of weight pouring down through the feet. Bend or take your knees down to your mat if you get tired.

Downward-Facing Dog with Blocks

Sometimes wrists get sore and we need to use tools such as blocks to alleviate the pressure on our wrists. Place the blocks wide on the mat, about an inch or so from the edge of the mat. Return to Tabletop Pose, with your hands on the blocks at the medium or lower height setting. If you choose the lowest height of the block, wrap your fingers around the top of the block. This hand placement changes the angle of your wrists and will help alleviate some wrist pain. From here, you can press back into Downward-Facing Dog.

Downward-Facing Dog with Forearms

This version of Downward-Facing Dog helps align, strengthen, and stretch the shoulders and can be useful for people who cannot bear weight on their wrists. Begin in Tabletop Pose. Now place your arms parallel to one another on the mat, with your elbows under your shoulders. Press down through your forearms and hug your elbows together energetically. Draw your shoulder blades together and curl your toes as you lift your hips up and back, distributing the weight evenly between your forearms and feet. If you feel that your head is too close to the ground, you can also place your forearms on blocks for this variation.

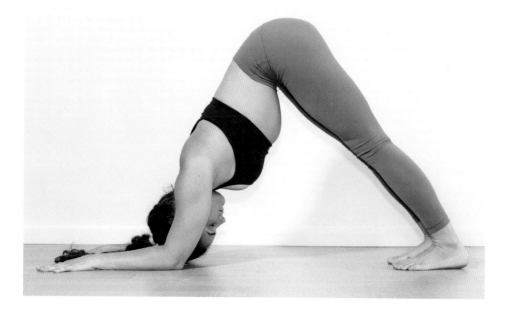

Sometimes modifying a pose isn't enough and instead it is recommended to practice another native. Child's Pose is used as a moment of deep inner reflection and often as a rest when even Downward-Facing Dog is too intense. Whether because of physical or emotional intensity, you will find great comfort in Child's Pose in your practice. Puppy Pose helps align and stretch the shoulders while providing a relief from the weight that can sometimes feel heavy in Downward-Facing Dog.

Puppy Pose / Uttana Shishosana

There are many ways to do *Uttana Shishosana*, or Puppy Pose. I recommend using a block if your shoulders are feeling tight. Extended Puppy Pose is a nice alternative to Downward-Facing Dog; I use it all the time. It is a combination of Downward-Facing Dog and Child's Pose, which is explained below.

Start from Tabletop Pose and release the tops of your feet down toward the mat. Walk your hands out in front of you, keep your arms engaged as you lower your chest down toward the mat, maintaining your upper body's connection to Downward-Facing Dog. Stay up on your fingers to activate your arms and keep lifting your elbows and forearms away from the ground. Draw your shoulder blades downward along your back and reach your hips toward your heels. You can place a block under your forehead to relieve neck stress.

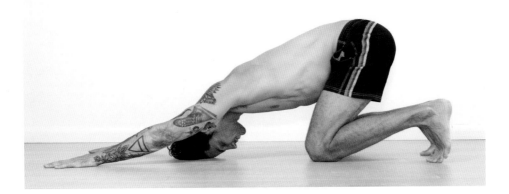

Child's Pose / Balasana

Start off in Tabletop Pose. Point your toes. Exhale as you gently shift your weight back to increase hip flexion. Settle your pelvis over your feet and fold your torso close to your thighs. Keep your arms extended outward and your elbows straight, if possible. Be careful not to externally rotate your hip joints or spread your knees too far apart. Ideally, hold your upper body onto your thighs. If you feel limited by your hip flexion, then place a bolster under your thighs. If you're using *Balasana*, or Child's Pose, as a rest from intense emotions, you may find it useful to soften your elbows and relax your shoulders.

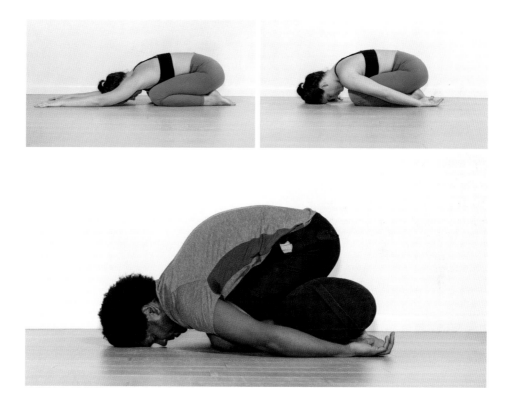

◆ ◆ ◆ ◆ ◆ ◆ ◆ ◆ ◆ ◆ ◆ ◆ ◆

Congratulations, you have now completed your first day of yoga challenge! The seeds of deep spiritual realization and personal growth and evolution are planted in the garden of your heart. Return to the practice tomorrow to continue your journey.

Plank Pose

Utthita Chaturanga Dandasana

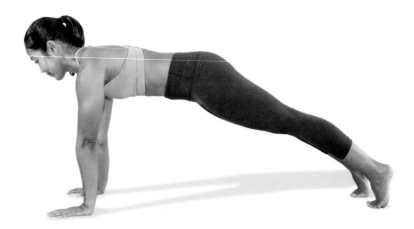

2

When I first started yoga, I was the weakest person in the room. There was just no way that I could have done the challenging asana that looks like a push-up. Now when I share yoga practice with students who, like me, struggle with strength, I always recommend starting off with Plank Pose, called *Utthita Chaturanga Dandasana* in Sanskrit because it is the most accessible version of Plank Pose I have found. Since the arms are straight, it is a bit easier to find healthy muscular and skeletal alignment without demanding too much upper-body strength from the start. Plank Pose allows students to build strength in all the right places with as much ease and comfort as is possible in an arm balance.

◆◆◆◆◆◆ ◆ ◆◆◆◆◆◆

Start off in Tabletop Pose to prepare for Plank Pose. Place your hands shoulder-width apart and your knees hip-width apart. Spread your fingers gently apart (but not to their maximum) and line up your index fingers with the inside edge of your wrists (parallel to the front of your mat). Curl your toes under and activate your feet. Widen your shoulder blades, round your upper back slightly, hug your ribs in toward the center of your body, and firm the muscles of your shoulder girdle. Straighten your arms while rooting down into the bases of your index fingers. Draw in your abdominal muscles of your abdomen toward your spine and tuck your tailbone to engage your lower abdominal muscles. Knit in the fibers of your entire torso and pelvic floor toward the centerline of your body to create a firm floor along the frontal portion of your body. Connect your legs into your pelvic floor and begin lifting your kneecaps and recruiting your quadriceps. Finally, inhale as you shift your shoulders slightly forward and lift up into Plank Pose. Check that your wrists are just around ninety degrees and grip your fingertips. Fold your ankles to a comfortable flexion and keep weight both in your toes and heels. Thrust with your arms and upper body into the ground while lifting up along the front side of your

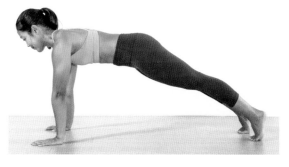

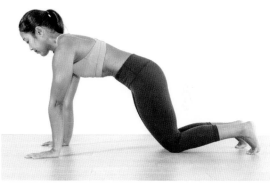

entire torso, from your ribs down to your pubic bone. Be very careful with your alignment to distribute the work of the pose to the strength of your abdomen, core, chest, shoulders, and arms. Keep your lower belly drawn deeply in and avoid overusing your back muscles. Gaze down to a single point between your hands just slightly ahead of your fingertips. Hold Plank Pose for at least one breath, then either transition down to a push-up, known as Chaturanga Dandasana, or return to your hands and knees and rest.

VARIATIONS

Plank Pose with Blocks

While Plank Pose is a relatively accessible pose for most, it can be really challenging if you have wrist pain, shoulder pain, or injuries, and/or you are working on building more upper-body strength. Creating variations for this pose helps everyone build strength and makes the practice accessible to all. Using blocks can help with wrist pain and shoulder pain while helping to build strength and body awareness.

Start in Tabletop Pose. Place your hands on blocks stacked about the width of the outer shoulder apart. Use the blocks on medium height and angled lengthwise toward the front of your mat. Grip the block to activate the muscles of your forearms. Press firmly into the blocks, straighten your arms, stack your shoulders over your wrists, and hug your elbows close to your body (but not touching). Apply all the instructions listed above to prepare. Then, as you inhale, firm your belly, tuck your tailbone, and extend one leg, keeping your toes curled under. If this feels comfortable and stable, extend your other leg and hug your inner thighs together while activating your quadriceps. Stay for at least one breath, then lower your knees back on your mat and rest. Or, for more advanced practitioners, lower into Chaturanga Dandasana with the support of the blocks and hover just above the ground.

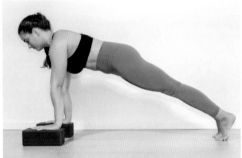 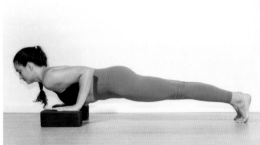

Advanced Plank Pose

Once you are established in Plank Pose, you might feel ready to transition to the more advanced Chaturanga Dandasana. I recommend not rushing into this. Many students start practicing Chaturanga Dandasana before their bodies are ready, and they end up predisposing themselves to avoidable injury. You know you're ready for Chaturanga Dandasana when you are comfortable in Plank Pose for at least five deep breaths.

To make this transition, start off in Plank Pose and slowly rotate the smiles of your elbows forward. This slight shift requires a lot of stabilization in the rotator cuff, so if you feel any instability while mobilizing your elbows here, I recommend not attempting Chaturanga Dandasana just yet. But if you're stable with that small shift of your elbows, then maintain all the strength and alignment detailed above and slowly bend your elbows while you lower your body toward the ground. Remember that Chaturanga Dandasana is still a plank pose and your body ideally stays knit together in one piece. Be extra conscious of tucking your tailbone and engaging the muscles of your lower abdomen to support your lumbar spine.

On the way into Chaturanga Dandasana, your shoulders and chest (particularly the pectorals major and minor) will need to activate even stronger. Go slowly. While the ideal alignment ends with your elbows at ninety degrees and your chest dipping down slightly under your arms, it takes years of practice to achieve this result. If this transition is too difficult, use one of the modifications listed below to build strength with healthy alignment.

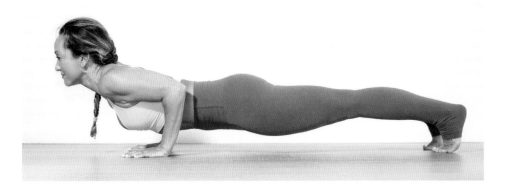

Plank Pose without Blocks on Knees

Students who lack the basic strength to maintain good alignment on the blocks and those who may be recovering from a shoulder injury would benefit from trying Plank Pose on their knees without blocks. From Tabletop Pose, take your hands out wide enough so that your outer shoulders line up with the centers of your wrists. Fully engage your hands with the pads of your fingers, pressing your knuckles down fully into the mat. Hug your forearms together and broaden your upper back. Keeping one or both knees down, shift your shoulders forward. Align your shoulders with your palms while keeping your belly engaged. Tuck your tailbone and keep your hips the same height as your shoulders.

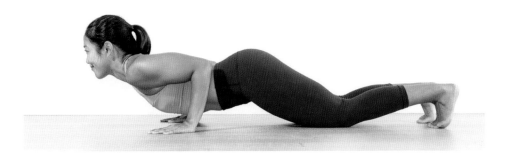

Using a Block or Bolster to Transition to Plank Pose

Bolsters are a great way to support your weight as you work on getting stronger.

Start from Tabletop Pose and place a block or bolster under your chest. Try experimenting with bolsters of different sizes or work with different sides and

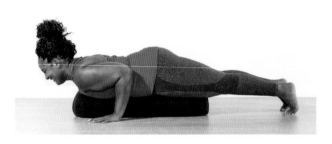

heights of your block. Bend your elbows and rest your sternum on the block or bolster, then extend your legs back. Firm your belly and then squeeze your legs together to create strength in the pose.

Plank Pose on the Floor

After you feel comfortable using the block or bolster to support your practice of Chaturanga Dandasana, you may be ready to try using the floor as a support for the pose.

Starting off in Utthita Chaturanga Dandasana, or Plank Pose, prepare to enter the bent-elbow push-up known as Chaturanga Dandasana in the manner outlined above. Instead of attempting to hover a few inches off the floor, simply aim to go all the way down to the ground so that your chest and thighs are supported by the ground. This floor-supported Chaturanga Dandasana is a great way to check your body's alignment. If your thighs remain elevated when you lower down, that is an indication that your pelvis is out of alignment. When you're on the floor, don't collapse. Instead, use the floor as a prop to help your body learn the structural integrity necessary to perform Chaturanga Dandasana. Maintaining a certain level of activa-

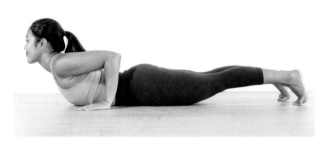

tion here is necessary to set up your body for transitioning out of this variation of the pose. As such, I recommend using the floor for support in Chaturanga Dandasana only for students who are proficient using the block or bolster option already.

Upward-Facing Dog

Urdhva Mukha Svanasana

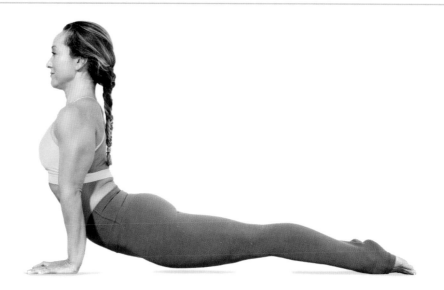

3

Backbending is a crucial part of yoga practice. As gravity affects the body over time and the aging process sets in, many of us literally get shorter as we get older. In fact, during the span of one day, the body is literally shorter by the end of the day. If you drive a car, you will notice this small shift by the adjustments you make in your rearview mirror by the end of the day. A night's rest is usually enough to rebalance the spine. But over time, unfortunately, gravity wins, and most people lose a bit of their height as they age. Along with this comes the predisposition to chronic back pain and other disorders related to spinal health. Backbending is a natural solution to this process. Not only are there physical benefits to backbending but also energetic, emotional, and even spiritual effects. As your spinal health returns, you can expect to feel your emotions more fully and enjoy increased vitality and mental alertness. What's wonderful about yoga practice is that you do not need to do contortion-style backbends to reap the benefits that backbends offer. Instead, a relatively accessible pose such as *Urdhva Mukha Svanasana*, or Upward-Facing Dog, opens the door for you to fully enjoy your practice and ultimately your life.

Start off in Plank Pose and gently shift your weight forward. Roll through your toes while keeping your ankles aligned with your shins (avoid rolling your ankles outward). Thrust into your arms to straighten your elbows. Release the tension in your abdominal wall needed for Plank Pose but keep your abdominal muscles pressed in toward your spine. Using your back muscles, begin to lift each joint of your spine, creating space between your ribs and hips. Release your tailbone, soften your glutes, and roll your thighs internally. Lift your thighs off the ground while keeping your lower back spacious. Expand your chest and lift your sternum. Elongate your neck and gaze toward your nose. Note that some advanced students will feel that their chest pops forward and pulls through the base of the arms. In this case, you can drop your head back onto the support of your trapezius muscles.

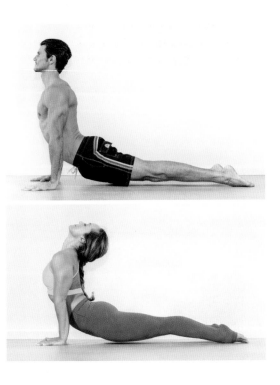

VARIATIONS
Upward-Facing Dog with a Bolster

Some students may find that Upward-Facing Dog is simply inaccessible. Whether due to a lack of spinal or wrist flexibility or other physical limitations, Upward-Facing Dog can be too demanding. Some curvy bodies may find that the dynamics often presupposed for the traditional pose simply do not work. Bigger bodies with bendy backs may even sometimes find Upward-Facing Dog ill-advised and uncomfortable. In all of these cases, using a bolster can really help if you don't feel strong enough to hold your weight on your hands or on the tops of your feet, or if your back simply does not have the flexibility yet.

Start in Tabletop Pose and place a bolster underneath your torso. Lower down slowly, drawing the lower tips of your shoulder blades down your back. Then lift your chest. Let your torso and legs rest on the bolster. Straighten your arms and press the tops of your feet down. Align your wrists, elbows, and shoulders on top of each other. In this posture, the weight of your body is positioned and supported on the bolster, which allows you to work on building strength. Gaze toward your nose and stay for at least one breath, but possibly up to five deep breaths. Exhale and roll into to Child's Pose or Downward-Facing Dog. Note that if you used blocks for any of the variations of Chaturanga Dandasana and Plank Pose you might consider keeping the blocks in place for Upward-Facing Dog as well.

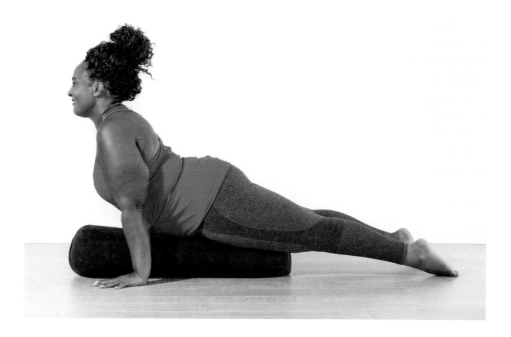

ALTERNATIVES TO UPWARD-FACING DOG

For some students, particularly those with very limited spinal extension and those with wrist injuries, lifting the body fully off the ground in Upward-Facing Dog will be too intense. In that case, it is recommended to practice an alternative to the pose.

Cobra Pose / Bhujangasana

Cobra Pose is a good alternative to Upward-Facing Dog if you cannot bear too much weight on your wrists, lack the strength to lift your body off the ground, or sometimes feel compression in your lower back when attempting Upward-Facing Dog.

Start off either in the floor-support variation of Chaturanga Dandasana or lie down on your stomach. Point your toes and activate the muscles of your legs. Stack your thighs in line with the outer edges of your hip joints and internally rotate your hips. Draw in your lower belly and lift your chest off the ground. Shift

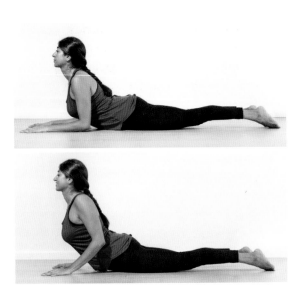

your elbows forward and bend your arms so that your elbows line up under your shoulders. Elevate your sternum as you root down through your elbows to create length and space through your upper back. Engage your back muscles to lift your chest and maximize the space between your ribs and hips. Elongate your neck (do not drop your head back) and lengthen your whole body, from the tips of your toes through the top of your head. If this feels comfortable, try lifting your elbows slightly off the ground to deepen the spinal extension.

If you have a hard time finding length through your back, try using a bolster under your rib cage to help lift your spine up and out of your pelvic bowl. Be mindful of compression sensations in your lower back and come down if you feel any pinching or sharp sensations. Gaze toward your nose and stay for at least one breath, but possibly up to five deep breaths. Exhale and roll into to Child's Pose or Downward-Facing Dog.

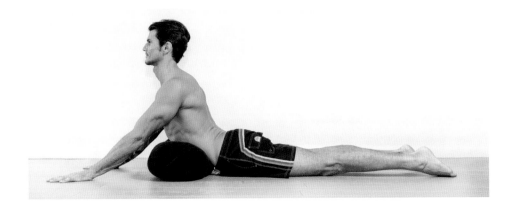

Upward-Facing Dog with Your Thighs on the Ground / High Cobra

This variation is a hybrid between Upward-Facing Dog and Cobra Pose, and it is great for students who find it impossible to keep their thighs off the ground while maintaining the spinal extension.

Modify the posture by employing all the alignments stated above but simply keep your thighs on the floor and bend your elbows slightly. Shift your hands forward of your shoulders to make space for the spinal extension. If you ever feel a crunching sensation in the joints of your spine you know that you're pushing too hard. Back off a little and find a variation of the pose that works for your body. And remember that your body is different every day!

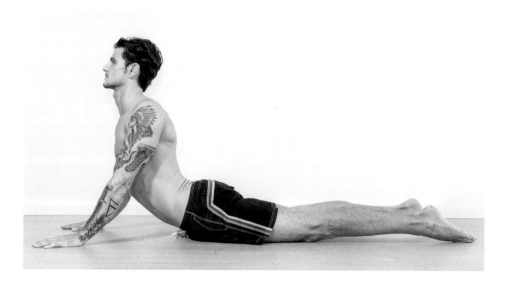

Chair Pose

Utkatasana

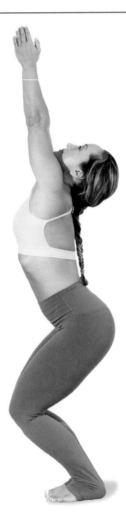

4

The simple act of getting up and down from a chair, sofa, car seat, or any other seated position is often one thing we take for granted until we lose our strength and flexibility. Practicing *Utkatasana*, Chair Pose, builds the basic strength and flexibility needed to maintain this basic function of the body while also laying the foundation for deeper, more challenging poses.

Start off by standing upright, leaving hands by your sides, also called *Samasthiti*. Align the bases of your big toes together. Root down through the bases of your big toes, your little toes, and your heels. Activate your pelvic floor and draw your lower abdominal muscles in toward your spine. Roll your thighbones toward each other to facilitate a gentle internal rotation of your hip joints. Allow your knees to bend slightly and angle together. Once your knees make contact with each other, engage your quadriceps while sending your femurs back into their sockets. Bend down a little more. Go gently, there is no need to drop your hips below your knees. Instead, focus on consciously activating all the muscles of your legs, pelvis, and torso. As you bend your knees, work in two directions—think about sending your femurs back while allowing your knees to come slightly forward. The action of sending your femurs back gives you access to the posterior portion of your hip sockets. This is the area where flexibility is often lost in old age and the area needed to maintain healthy function of the hips, including standing up and sitting down. Do not take your knees too far beyond your toes or you may lose the grounding through your heels. Your thighs should burn somewhat from the engagement. Maintain a deep steady breath. Notice the muscular sensation but try not to identify with it or let it deter you from practicing deeply.

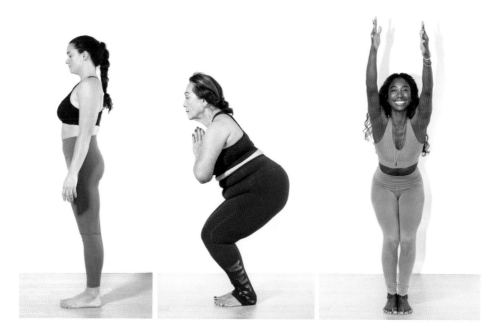

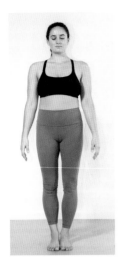

Next, once your legs are in place, begin to actively lift your ribs away from your hips along all sides of the body equally. Avoid arching your back. Instead, allow your tailbone to be heavy and weighted but not tucked. Take your hands in prayer position, resting your thumbs at the center of your chest. Gaze toward your nose. Stay for a few breaths. If you feel comfortable, gently extend your arms forward. Drop your shoulder blades down your back so that you feel your shoulders rolling open to give space to your neck. Focus on straightening your elbows completely and let your hands point in whatever direction your shoulder mobility allows, rather than pointing your fingers up toward the ceiling. Gaze toward your thumbs. Stay for at least five breaths. Then straighten your legs, drop your arms down by your sides, and return to Samasthiti.

VARIATIONS
Chair Pose with a Wide Stance

Chair Pose builds strength in the legs but can often be too challenging for bigger bodies or students with bad balance. To make this pose more accessible and comfortable for all, try taking your feet wider apart. Think about setting your feet either hip-width or the width of a yoga block apart, or potentially even wider.

Start off in Samasthiti and spread your feet to around hip-width apart. Find the stance where you feel most comfortable. Keep your weight evenly distributed between both feet and align your knees over your feet. Do not try to draw your knees toward each other as stated in the alignment pointers above. You can work with a very gentle internal rotation of your hip joints, but be sure that your knees track forward in line with your feet. Keep your back as flat as possible and activate your core muscles to support your spine. Hinging at your waist while keeping a flat back and resting your torso on your thighs can also be helpful for beginners and older students. When working with your arm position, start off with your hands in prayer position at your heart-center. Then extend your arms into "goal post" arms or "cactus" arms to make the full shoulder extension more accessible. Concentrate on externally

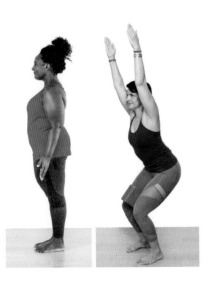

rotating your shoulders and avoid taking your arms apart too wide. If your shoulders are sore, try placing your elbows on your knees instead of extending your arms upward.

Chair Pose with a Wide Stance and a Block

Sometimes it can be hard to feel or activate your legs; other times it can be difficult to balance. In either case, placing a yoga block between your legs when you practice Utkatasana with the wider stance can be really helpful.

Start off in Samasthiti and spread your feet to about hip-width apart. Place the block between your knees, finding the position of the block that works best for your stance. Root down into the bases of your big toes, little toes, and heels. Be sure that your knees track in line with your feet. Gently squeeze the block by activating the muscles of your inner your thighs and drawing your legs together in the motion called "adduction" and rotating your hip joints inward. Follow the directions outlined above. The benefit of adding the block to Utkatasana is that you now have a very real tactile sense of where your legs are. If you do not activate your legs, the block will fall down. This added activation helps firm your thighs, increase your sense of balance and the placement of your body in space, called proprioception, and make this pose even more accessible.

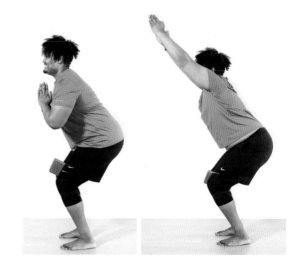

Chair Pose with a Chair

Some people will simply not be able to access Utkatasana from standing. Whether you are older, recovering from an injury or brain trauma, or simply not feeling well, you can always try Chair Pose from a chair!

Choose a hard-backed chair, such as a dining chair or office chair, and sit down comfortably. Be sure that your feet touch the ground when your hips are snuggled into the chair. Scoot slightly forward so that your hips rest on the edge of the seat. Align your feet and knees either together or about hip-width apart. Begin to root down into the bases of your big toes, little toes, and your heels.

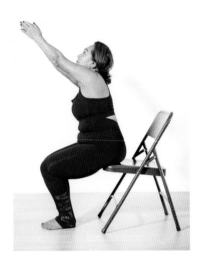

Activate your pelvic floor and draw your lower abdominal muscles in toward your spine. Keeping your back as flat as possible, pivot forward through your hip joints and lean forward. Leave your hands on the seat of the chair. Allow your neck to follow your spine and avoid looking up. Stay for a few breaths. If you're comfortable, bring your hands to prayer position at your heart-center and eventually work up to extending your arms up in cactus position or with your palms pressed together. Finally, if you feel the weight in your legs and the strength in your body, gently rock forward and lift your hips a few inches off the chair. Stay for five breaths. Return to your seat.

Chair Pose with the Wall

Stand with your back facing the wall. Back up to the wall closely, so that your back is resting flat against the wall. Keep your feet about a foot away from the wall. Root down into the bases of your big toes, little toes, and heels. Activate your pelvic floor and draw the lower abdominal muscles in toward your spine. Keeping

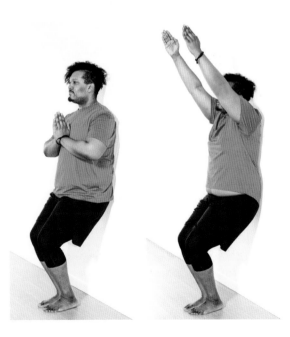

your back as flat as possible, press your lower back into the wall. Keep your hands by your sides. Find the stance where you feel most comfortable, feet and knees together or feet hip-width apart. Keep your weight evenly distributed between both feet and align your knees over your feet. Gently bend your knees while sliding your back down the wall. Leave your hands by your sides or take your hands to prayer position. Stay for five breaths. Slide back up the wall and return to standing.

Wide-Legged Forward Fold

Prasarita Padottanasana

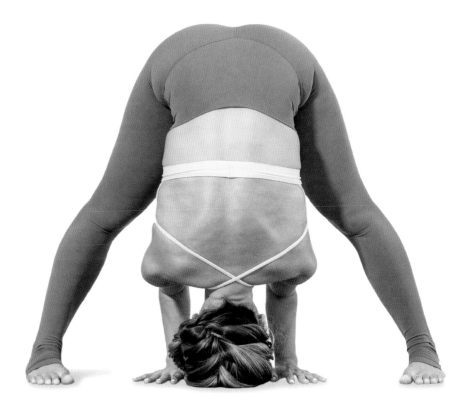

5

Wide-Legged Forward Fold is one of the most accessible standing forward folds in yoga practice. Since the feet are wider apart, it makes the forward bending easier for most people. The distance between the feet is somewhat adjustable, making this pose even more adaptable than most. As with all standing forward folds, gravity helps you find the lift through your inner body. There is a natural emptiness in your pelvic bowl as your organs are encouraged to float up into your thoracic cavity. This change of perspective can sometimes create dizziness, so it is important to remember to breathe deeply as you enter and exit the pose.

Start in Samasthiti. Then inhale and step your feet wide apart. Again, this varies depending on your height, leg length, and flexibility. If you feel tighter, then step your feet as wide apart as possible. If you feel more flexible, you might be able to step only a slight width apart. Either way, keep your weight evenly distributed between both feet. Allow a very slight turning of your toes inward so that the outer edges of your feet are lined up with the bases of your little toes. It's easy to turn your feet outward here, so watch your foot alignment. Activate your inner thighs and draw your legs in toward each other. Lift the arches of your feet and activate the muscles that control your ankles. Gently place your hands on your waist. Inhale as you lift your ribs away from your hips, activate your pelvic floor, and pull the lower abdominal muscles in toward your spine. Exhale as you fold forward, pivoting from your hips, and aim your hands down toward the ground.

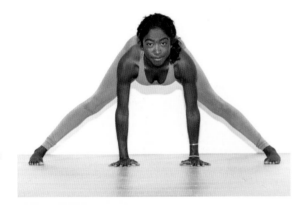

Lift your sitting bones away from your heels while extending the full length of your hamstrings and backs of your legs. Line up your fingers and toes and keep your hands flat and shoulder-width apart. Look forward and slightly up as you inhale. Exhale and fold your torso down between your thighs. Pivot even deeper into the inner space of your pelvis and allow your gluteal muscles to release and spread ever so slightly apart. Relax your back and aim the top of your head toward the floor. Gaze toward your nose. Stay for five breaths. Inhale, lift your torso halfway up, straighten your arms, and exhale there. Inhale as you shift your hands to your waist and come all the way back up to standing. Exhale and return to Samasthiti.

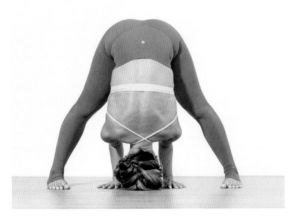

Wide-Legged Forward Fold with Blocks

If your fingertips don't quite reach the floor, this can be a very difficult pose. Spreading your feet too wide apart is not an option because you will feel as though you are collapsing onto the floor. Using blocks will help stabilize you in the posture.

Set up in the manner outlined above, and then place two blocks where your hands would touch the floor, and one block where your head would touch the floor. When you fold forward, aim for the blocks instead of the floor. If your hands touch the floor, then place one block on the floor where your head would make contact. Bend from your hips and lean forward, pointing the crown of your head down. Exhale as you place the top of your head on the block. Keep your weight held in your pelvic floor and grounded down through your legs.

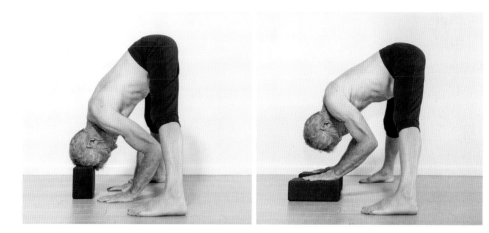

Wide-Legged Forward Fold with the Wall

If yoga blocks are not available to you, or if you're recovering from a back injury or your balance is challenged, you might find it easier to use the wall for support and refrain from going all the way down to the ground. Using the wall allows your back to find extra support and helps make space for bigger torsos.

Stand facing the wall, with your feet spread widely apart and your hands on your waist. Follow the same preparations outlined above. Exhale as you take your hands to the wall, placing your palms flat against the wall. Your body will remain at approximately ninety degrees. Pivot even deeper into the inner space of your pelvis and allow your gluteal muscles to release and spread ever so slightly apart.

Relax your back and aim the crown of your head toward the floor. Gaze toward your nose. Stay for five breaths. Inhale, lift your torso halfway up, straighten your arms, and exhale there. Inhale as you shift your hands to your waist and come all the way back up to standing. Exhale and return to Samasthiti.

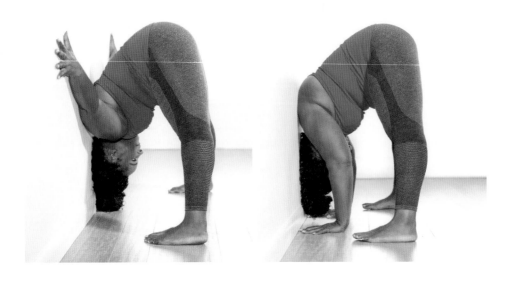

Triangle Pose
Trikonasana

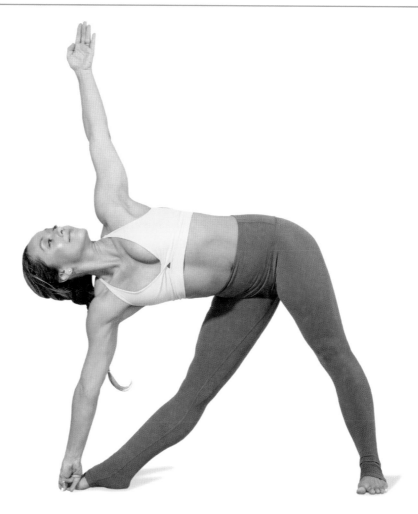

6

Trikonasana, or Triangle Pose, is a foundational asana that builds strength, flex-ibility, alignment, and awareness. Despite its relative ease, it is not by any means easy. Trikonasana is also a challenging balancing pose for any students who may not be stable on their legs. It's important to break down the anatomical pointers so that you can practice safely and confidently. Let's get started.

Start in Samasthiti. Then inhale and step your feet about three to four feet apart. This varies depending on your height, leg length, and flexibility. Spread your arms out to your sides so that they parallel the floor and form a T. Externally rotate your right hip joint and turn your right foot out to the side ninety degrees. Root down into the bases on your big toes, little toes, and heels. Allow your arches to lift as you activate your quadriceps and inner thighs. It should feel almost as though you are squeezing your thighs toward each other and adducting your thighs.

Draw in your lower belly toward your spine and activate your pelvic floor. Locate your hips, hip joints, and the area around your right hip crease. Exhale as you pivot into the right hip joint and allow your torso to slide over to the side. Be careful not to just do a side bend from your ribs. Instead, allow your hips to shift slightly toward the left and use the space to fold your torso in toward your right hip joint. Avoid arching or rounding your spine. Align your shoulders with your hips.

Glide your right hand toward your right foot and wrap your thumb, index finger, and middle finger around your big toe. If you are unable to reach your toe but you feel stable in your legs, then you might find it more accessible to allow your fingertips to hover on the outer edges of your shin. Avoid pushing down with your right hand into your shin. Reach your left hand up toward the ceiling and gaze toward your left fingers. Stack your shoulders in line with each other and keep your chest broad. Stay for five breaths, then come up and switch sides.

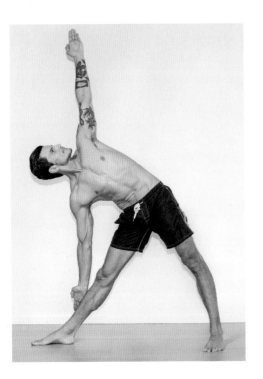

If you are new to the practice, you may want to place extra emphasis on strengthening your knees in Trikonasana. Distribute your weight as evenly as possible between your feet. If you feel any discomfort in the back of your knees, try rooting down more powerfully into the bases of your big toes. Avoid dumping weight into your knees. If the pain persists, then consider shortening your stance.

Triangle Pose with a Block

Using a block for a little extra support in Trikonasana helps immensely with balance and stability. Not everyone will be able to grab their toes in the pose, but with the help of a block everyone can find a sense of deep grounding.

To enter Trikonasana with the block, place the block on the outside of your right foot. Then, following the same instructions outlined above, instead of reaching toward your big toe, place your fingertips or your flat palm on the block when you go down. Reach your left hand up toward the ceiling and gaze toward your left fingers. Stack your shoulders in line with each other and keep your chest broad. Stay for five breaths, then come up and switch sides.

Triangle Pose for Sore Shoulders

For some students, extending their arms fully can be quite painful. If your shoulders are sore or injured, try placing your left hand on your waist instead of extended outward. Or try grabbing your elbows behind your back. Release the neck muscles and gaze slightly up and toward the left.

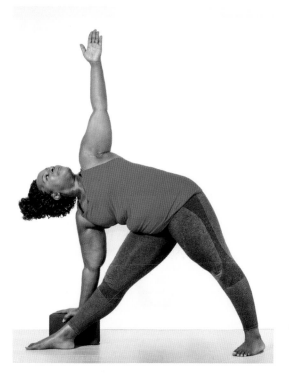

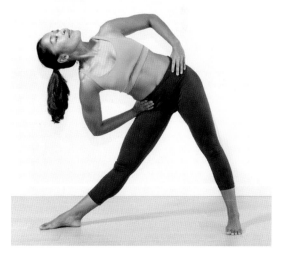

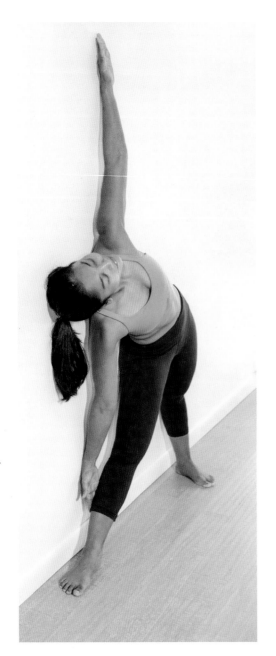

Triangle Pose with the Wall

For students with bad balance or those
wishing to test the alignment of their hips,
using a wall is a great tool for practice.

Start off with your back facing the wall.
Keep your butt and shoulders as close
to the wall as possible. If your balance is
challenged, then try leaning against the
wall for stability. Following the directions
outlined above, enter Trikonasana. You
will most likely not be able to grab your
toe, nor should you try. Instead, focus on
the inner work of the pose.

Crane Pose

Bakasana

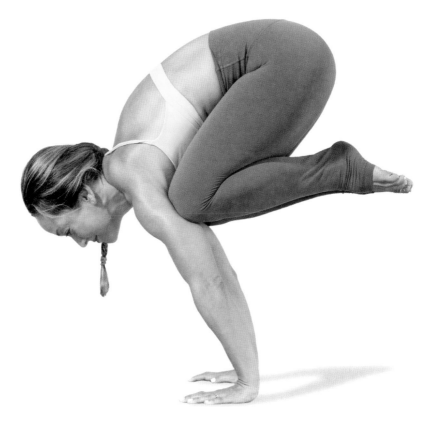

7

The lesson of arm balances is often about strength and self-confidence. Remember, this isn't a competition, and you are not being judged by how high you lift up. Instead, the journey into *Bakasana*, or Crane Pose, is about finding spiritual strength. This arm balance is a combination of strength and flexibility. When I first started, I used to slide off my arms all the time. But each time I slid down or tumbled out, I got back up again just that little bit stronger. If you find yourself unable to lift up or you fall out almost immediately after entering Bakasana, pick yourself back up again and know that you're getting stronger each time. Don't give up.

The truth is that Bakasana can be a really difficult pose for a lot of students. It can be especially challenging if you have a larger body or you are not naturally strong. Some of the things that might keep you from executing this pose efficiently include too much pressure on wrists, fear of falling forward, or the inability to get your knees high enough on your elbows to find balance. You may feel unstable on your arms and intimidated by this arm balance. Just go slowly and give yourself ample time to build strength. You will cultivate both patience and forbearance along the way.

• • • • • • ◆ • • • • • •

Start off in Downward-Facing Dog. Step forward to a deep squat. Keep your feet together and spread your knees apart. Slide your torso down between your

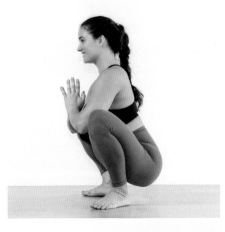

thighs. Place your hands on the ground, shoulder-width apart. Allow your elbows to bend slightly and point back, but avoid splaying your arms out to the side. Root down into the bases of your index fingers while gripping with all of your fingertips. Keep the heels of your hands pressed firmly down. Stack your knees either on your triceps, on the outer edges of the arms close to your shoulders, or in your armpits. Firm your shoulders and stabilize your entire shoulder girdle. Round your back and activate your abdominal muscles. Recruit your transverse abdominals to knit your torso together. Come forward onto the balls of your feet and pour weight forward into your shoulders. Press into the ground with the strength of your shoulders. Inhale as you send your chest forward and lift your hips slightly back and up. Find the counterbalance point where lift-off happens. Try lifting one foot and then the other. Or try lifting both feet at the same time.

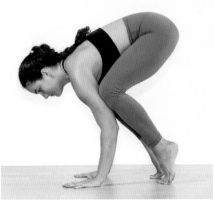

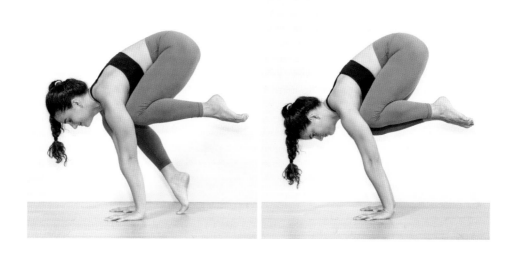

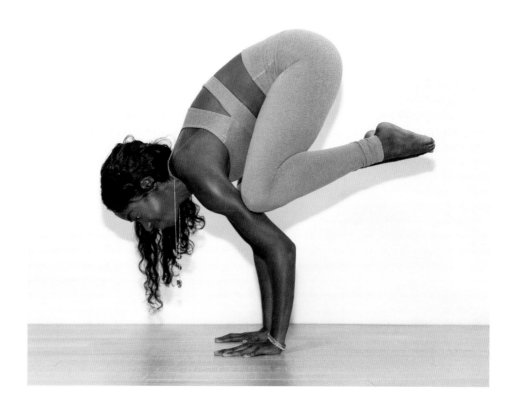

Reclining Crane

If you find Bakasana to be inaccessible or you want to try a creative variation, try it on your back. Lie on your back and bring your knees into your chest. Bring your big toes together, point your feet, and spread your knees wide apart. Draw your lower ribs toward your hips and activate your abdominal muscles as you bring your

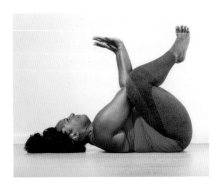

elbows to the inside of your knees. Press your palms into the air. Adjust your feet so that the inner edges of your feet press together and your lower ribs press into your mat. This achieves the basic shape of Crane Pose without placing weight in your arms, hands, or wrists. And what's more, it gives you the feeling of Bakasana while building the muscular strength you need to one day achieve the full pose. Stay for five breaths, then come down.

Crane on a Block

Use a block to help you position your knees higher on the backs of your arms and elevate your feet into a more lifted position. Step up onto one or two blocks and come into wide-legged squat. Bring your knees wide apart and place your hands flat on the mat. Lean forward as you engage your inner thighs and push from your shoulders through your arms. Hug your elbows in slightly toward each other to avoid splaying your elbows out to your sides. Press your knees gently into your arms to activate muscle tension in your core. Continue leaning forward gently until your feet lift off the block. Play with lifting one leg off the floor at a time. If you need extra height, try placing both hands on blocks in the same manner outlined above for Plank Pose. Stay for five breaths, then come down.

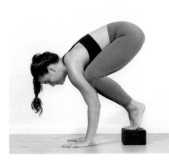
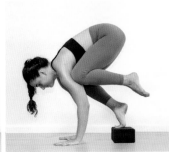
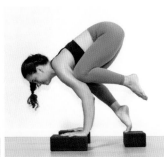

Crane with the Wall

A more daring variation is to play with Crane Pose at the wall. Begin in a very low squat, with your back to the wall, your knees wide, and your toes turned out. Once you feel comfortable in this position, place your hands on the floor or on blocks in the lowest height setting. Lean forward and bring your knees toward your triceps as you press from your shoulders and pour weight into your hands. Step one foot up the wall and then the other. This variation is good to try for students of all levels. Advanced students may think about entering from a wall plank position. If you feel unstable, try placing your head on a block and press down firmly on the block with your forehead. If you feel strong enough, lift your head away from the block by pressing down into your hands and feet. Stay for five breaths, then come down.

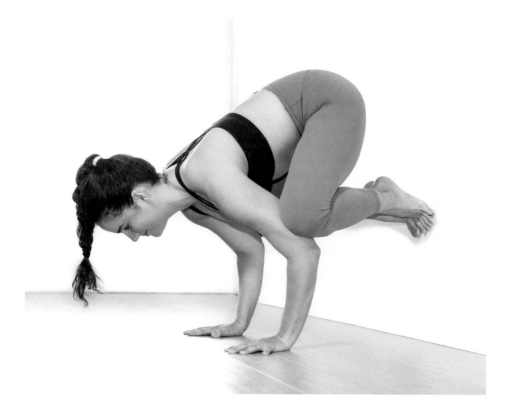

Butterfly Pose
Baddha Konasana

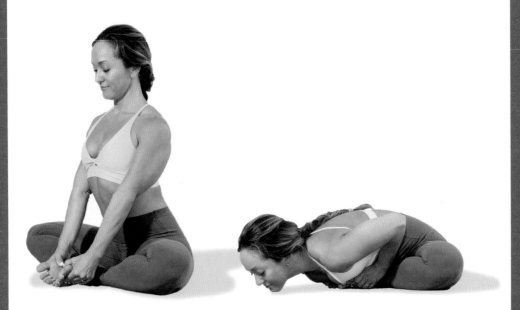

Tightness along the inner thighs is an impediment to the external rotation on which so many yoga poses rely. Similarly, stiff legs often result from stress or trauma and can signal less than optimal bodily health. *Baddha Konasana* has many English names that refer to it, including Butterfly Pose, Bound Angle Pose, or Cobbler's Pose, all of which are acceptable. This pose targets the inner thighs in an effort to free up access to the hips. While the dynamics of the pose make it generally accessible to different body types, it is by no means easy. In fact, Baddha Konasana can be quite demanding from a physical and emotional perspective. The hips are the seat of deep emotions, and it is not uncommon to be flooded with emotions, memories, or other feelings in the body when practicing Baddha Konasana. If you find this happens to you while practicing this pose, you are on the right track. If not, don't worry, keep practicing.

You never need to endure physical pain during your yoga practice. However, you shouldn't be afraid of muscular burning sensations. Always keep your joints safe and protected, and never push through burning sensations around your joints. In a pose such as Baddha Konasana, it is rather common to experience discomfort along your inner thighs and lower back. Be sure that your knee joints are not under stress in this or any yoga pose.

Start off in a comfortable seated position, then gently place the soles of your feet together. Draw your heels in as close to your groin as possible. Close your knee joints and seal your calf muscles and inner thighs together as much as possible. Gently wrap your hands around the outer edges of your feet. Place the tips of your thumbs under the mounds of your big toes. Activate your feet by pressing the outer edges of your little toes and the outer edges of your heels into each other. Lift the soles of your feet upward. Tune in to your greater trochanters on the outer edges of your thighbones and send them back and away from each other to facilitate external rotation. The movement dynamic created by externally rotating the hip joints encourages an opening of the feet and a spreading of the knees. Engage your pelvic floor. Keep your spine and arms straight and your sitting bones on the ground. Gaze toward your nose. Stay for five breaths.

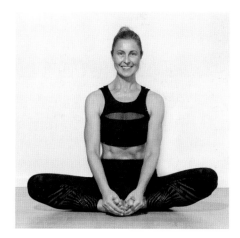

If you feel comfortable, you might consider folding forward. Treat this as any forward bend and initiate the action of the movement from deep within your pelvis. Drawing in your lower belly, pivot from behind your pubic bone. Keep your back as straight as possible while sending your chest forward. Once you reach a limit, allow your back to round slightly and place your forehead or chin on the ground. If you cannot comfortably fold forward, you might simply leave your head floating in the air.

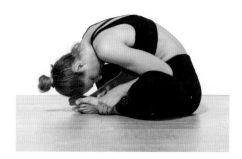

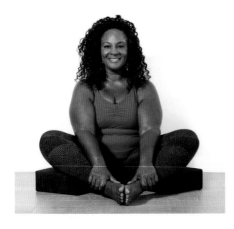

VARIATION
Butterfly Pose with Blocks

If there is excessive pulling in your inner hip muscles or strain on your knees, place blocks underneath each of your knees. Try angling each block so that the flat part presses into your outer thigh. Another variation for this pose is to place a block between the soles of your feet to create more space. Pressing your feet into the block allows you to root more firmly into your sitting bones. In this variation, you might find that it is better to simply sit upright with your hands on blocks. Finally, when you fold forward, if you are very far away from the ground, you might find it helpful to place your hands or your head on a block for additional support.

ALTERNATIVES TO BUTTERFLY POSE
Reclining Butterfly Pose / Supta Baddha Konasana

Trying a different entry may help you access the inner thighs more deeply. Any reclining pose offers you the chance to really dive inward and explore your body from a meditative point of awareness. Start off lying flat on your back, legs extended on your mat and along your sides. Bend your knees, place the soles of your feet on the floor, and draw your knees together. Externally rotate your hips, activate your pelvic floor, and allow your knees to drop down by your sides. Place blocks or bolsters under your knees for additional support, as needed. If lying flat creates stress in your lower back, try lying over a bolster. If your feet slide out, try tying a strap around your feet and anchoring the strap gently around your hips. Stay for ten to twenty breaths. Close your eyes.

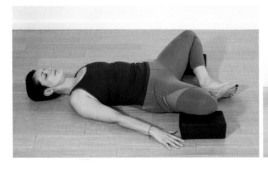

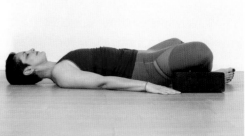

Happy Baby Pose / Ananda Balasana

Happy Baby Pose is a good alternative pose for Baddha Konasana because it achieves a similar shape and may be more accessible for some people.

Starting on your back, draw your knees into your chest. Hold the back of your thighs as you open your knees and flex your feet up to the sky. Clasp your ankles, the outer edges of your feet, or the backs of your thighs. If you are comfortable, try bringing the soles of your feet together in the shape of Butterfly Pose.

Another option is to take a strap and place it around the knuckles of your toes, bringing your feet up and out. Happy Baby Pose can also be done with one leg at a time. Try looping the strap around your leg to draw it in, or grabbing the side of your foot and bringing your knee toward the outer edge of your rib cage.

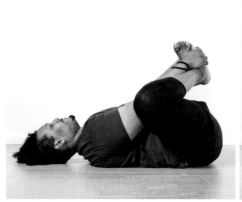 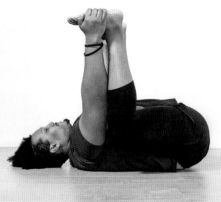

Extended Side Angle Pose

Utthita Parsvakonasana A

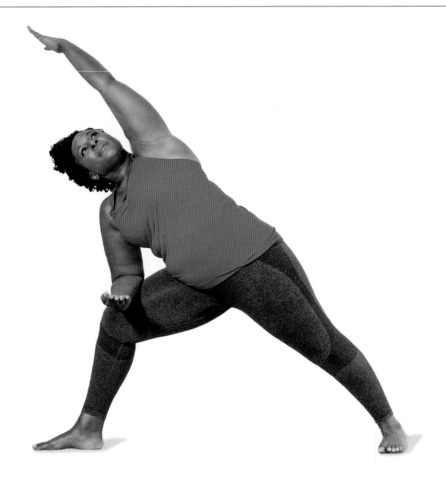

9

As a foundational asana, *Utthita Parsvakonasana* A, or Extended Side Angle Pose, offers insight into so many fundamental movements in yoga practice. You will find leg strengthening, hip rotation, core work, and shoulder articulation. The inner energetics of this pose ask you to ground down through your legs while simultaneously lifting powerfully upward. Utthita Parsvakonasana A helps with balance and emotional stability, and it energizes and cleanses the body. This pose can easily be made accessible for all body types.

Start off in Samasthiti. Inhale as you take a wide step out to the right. Activate your inner thighs as though you are drawing your legs in toward each other, but maintain the wide-legged stance. Lift the arches of your feet and activate the muscles that control your ankles. Spread your arms up and out to your sides so that they parallel the floor in a T-shape. Externally rotate your right hip joint and turn your right foot out to the side ninety degrees. Root down into the bases on your big toes, little toes, and heels. Allow your arches to lift as you activate your quadriceps and inner thighs. Draw in your lower belly toward your spine and activate your pelvic floor.

Locate your hip joints and the area around your right hip crease. Bend your right knee down over your right ankle and feel the solidity of your legs. Slowly begin to fold your torso over to the right. Glide down toward your right hip joint. Exhale as you hook your right forearm on your right inner thigh. Roll your left shoulder externally as you extend your left arm in line with the left side of your body. Gaze toward your left fingers. Stay for five breaths. Then switch to the other side.

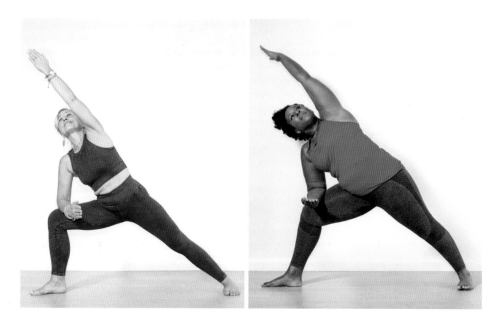

To move deeper, dangle your right hand along the outer edge of your right thigh. Allow your fingertips to graze the floor or rest firmly on the ground.

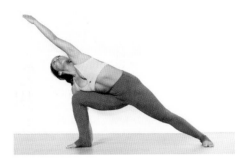

Once your fingers root down on the ground, allow your torso to slide around the thigh. Line up your fingers with your foot. Maintain the same alignment as above. Avoid arching your back or bending forward to try to force your fingers down. If your fingers are comfortably down, then press the whole hand firmly down.

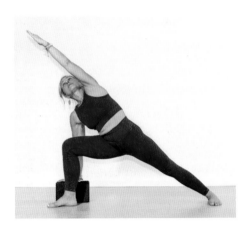

Extended Side Angle Pose with a Block

If you find that resting your forearm on your thigh is too easy but touching the floor is too hard, try using a block. Place the block on the outer edge of your right foot. Then, following the instructions outlined above, place your hand or your right fingertips on the block to enter Utthita Parsvakonasana A.

Extended Side Angle Pose with a Chair

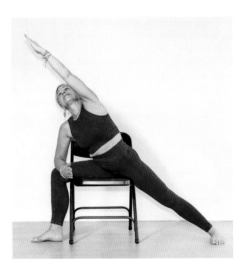

Start off sitting on a chair. Your feet should comfortably touch the floor with both soles flat and your thighs should be parallel with the ground. Slide forward to the edge of the chair and activate your pelvic floor. Externally rotate out your right hip joint while reaching to the side with your left leg. Hook your right forearm on your right inner thigh and extend your left arm. Follow the alignment pointers outlined above. Use the chair for added stability and try to lift your weight off the chair. Hold the pose with your weight lifted off the chair for an additional one to three breaths and then return to seated position.

Locust Pose

Shalabhasana

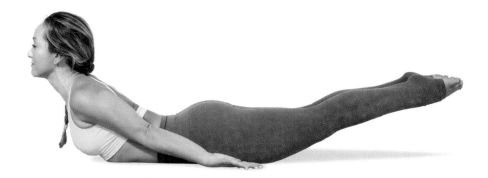

10

A healthy spine increases energy and vitality. Backbending is key to the health of the spine, and in yoga it's wonderful when you start identifying backbends that your body can safely enter. Shalabhasana, or Locust Pose, is one of the most beneficial and accessible poses in yoga practice. In this pose you can expect to strengthen your back muscles deeply. This type of work may be challenging at first, but if you stick with it, Shalabhasana can be therapeutic for all sorts of back pain.

◆◆◆◆◆◆ ◆ ◆◆◆◆◆◆

Start by lying face down on your mat, in a prone position. Place your forehead on the floor. Align your arms by your sides and set the tops of the hands on the ground. Touch the bases of your big toes together and gently roll your hip joints internally. Activate your pelvic floor and draw your abdominal muscles in toward your spine. Lift your kneecaps up to engage the quadriceps. Gently lift your legs by sending your thighs back and up. Do not worry about how high

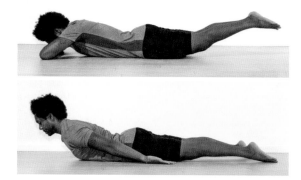

you lift your legs off the ground. Instead, think about elongating the muscles and joints of your back. Send your rib cage up and forward while maximizing the space between your ribs and hips. Roll your shoulders forward and gently press your fingertips into the ground. Avoid craning your neck back; instead, reach out through

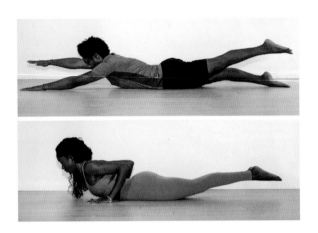

the top of your head. It is tempting to squeeze your glutes, but this is actually counterproductive to the inner work of backbending. If you attempt to squeeze your glutes to lift your legs, you will push your pubic bone into the ground and flatten your lower back. Instead, focus on lengthening your back and extending out with your legs. Gaze toward your nose. Stay for five breaths.

VARIATION
Locust Pose with a Bolster

Even though Locust Pose is relatively accessible, it can be very challenging if you are unable to hold a lot of weight on the front part of your body. For example, if you're pregnant, or have a larger chest or midsection, it might not be advised to lie on your stomach. Try placing a bolster underneath your hip bones to lessen the amount of weight placed on the front of your body.

Start by lying face down with your forehead on the mat. Extend your arms out in front of you and your legs straight back behind you. Lift your legs only as high as possible while continuing to draw your thighs together. For another variation, begin by lying face down on your mat with your arms stretched out

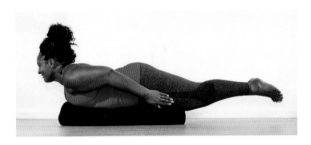

in front of you and your legs stretched out behind you. Press your legs down into the mat and start squeezing your thighs together. Then lift only your upper body off the mat. Draw the lower tips of your shoulder blades down your back.

Tiger Pose or Leg Lifts

This variation is recommended for pregnant women and anyone else who is not advised to place any weight on their midsection, such as those recovering from abdominal surgery. Start off in Tabletop Pose. Extend your spine. Gently lift your left leg by sending it back and up. Drop your left hip and align your foot, ankle, and hip joint. Keep your pelvic floor and lower belly drawn in. Stay for a few breaths.

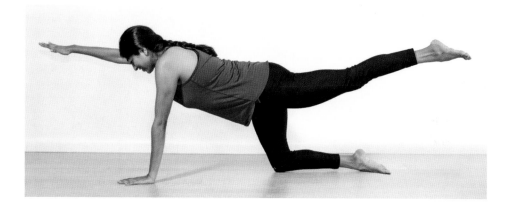

Next, lift your right leg and your left arm. Think about creating as much length and space as possible between the joints of your spine. Gaze down and slightly forward. For a challenge, try Tiger Pose, *Eka Hasta Vyaghrasana*. Bend your right leg, reach back with your left hand, and grab your right ankle. If you cannot reach, don't force it.

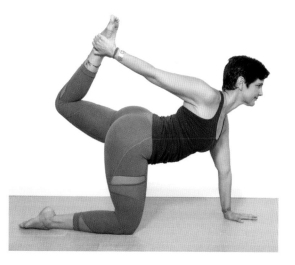

Simple Bridge Pose
Sukha Setu Bandhasana

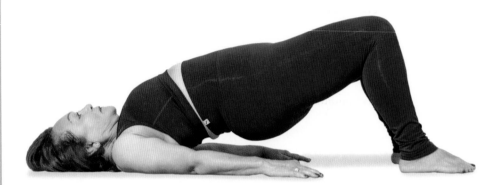

11

Backbending awakens all the energy centers, or chakras, along the spine. You don't need to believe in esoteric philosophies to feel the effect. As soon as you start backbending, you will feel a strong sensation of heat rise up from your core. This powerful force brings vital life flow, or prana, into your mind and body. You may feel charged up after backbends. Or you may also feel tired. It really just depends on how your system responds to the new influx of energy.

◆ ◆ ◆ ◆ ◆ ◆ ◆ ◆ ◆ ◆ ◆ ◆ ◆

Start by lying on your back with both knees bent and the soles of your feet flat on the floor. Align your knees and feet with the outer edges of your hips. Slide your arms alongside your body. Press the backs of your arms and the soles of your feet into the floor. Activate your pelvic floor and draw your navel in toward your spine. Lift your rib cage away from your hips and begin to extend your spine.

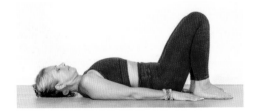

Think about your sternum rising up and touching your chin. Firm your quadriceps and send your hips forward and up. Slowly roll your spine away from the floor, starting with your pelvis, to come up into *Sukha Setu Bandhasana*, or Simple Bridge Pose. Gaze toward your nose. Stay for five breaths.

If you're ready to go a bit deeper, interlace your fingers under your hips. If this feels easy, try wrapping your hands around your ankles to prepare. Then inhale and lift up into Simple Bridge Pose, following the instructions outlined above. Gaze toward your nose. Stay for five breaths.

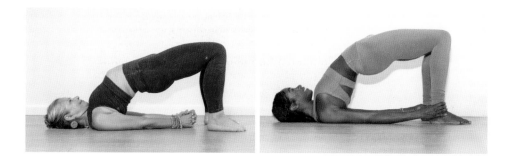

VARIATIONS
Simple Bridge Pose for Bigger Bodies
If catching your ankles or interlacing your fingers is not possible, spread your hands wider apart and, if using a yoga mat, you might even grab the edges of your mat with your hands. Think about spreading your arms apart and pulling the mat apart as if you're trying to stretch the mat wider. This action may give you more leverage to lift your hips higher.

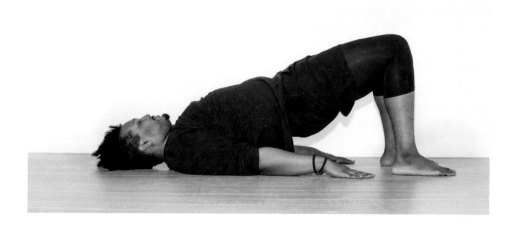

Simple Bridge Pose with a Block

If you have a hard time lining up your feet, knees, and thighs, and your knees tend to splay out to the sides, try using a block. Place a block between your thighs and squeeze your knees together. This action encourages the correct muscular work needed to set up the pose. Maintaining the muscular activation around the block, inhale to lift up into Simple Bridge Pose.

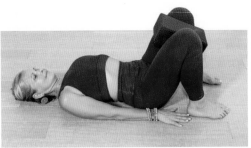

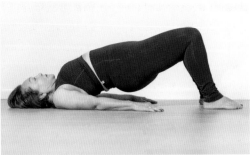

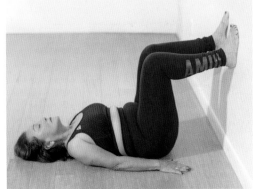

Simple Bridge Pose with a Wall

If you find it very difficult to lift your hips, practice Simple Bridge Pose while using the wall for support. Start with your legs up the wall. Then bend the knees and press the soles of your feet into the wall as your lift your hips away from the ground.

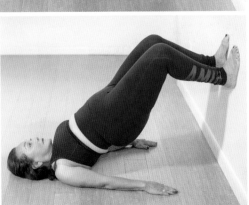

Upward-Facing Bow Pose / Urdhva Dhanurasana

Once you feel stable in Simple Bridge Pose, you might be ready to try *Urdhva Dhanurasana*, or Upward-Facing Bow Pose. After some time practicing Simple Bridge Pose, your body may be encouraging you toward a natural and useful progression to deepen your spinal extension and begin working this slightly more challenging backbend. As the arms are extended over the head there is a greater demand placed on the shoulders and upper back. Don't rush into this backbend; instead, really put in the work in Simple Bridge Pose.

To prepare, lie on your back. Bend your knees and align your feet hip-width apart. Bend your elbows and place your hands under your shoulders. Align your elbows with your shoulders. Engage the muscles of your pelvic floor, root down into your feet, and inhale as you roll onto the top of your head. You might choose to stay here or, if you can breathe and your body feels good, you might feel ready to lift up all the way into Urdhva Dhanurasana.

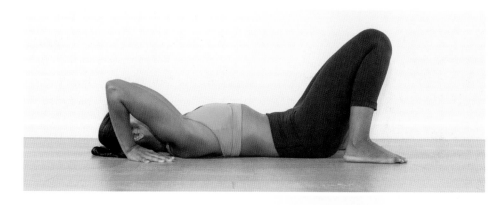

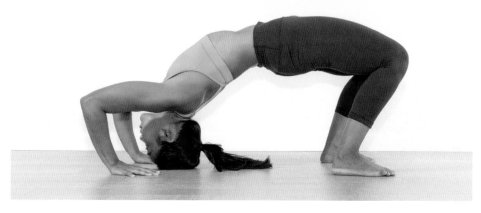

Following the same instructions outlined above to lift up into Simple Bridge Pose, all you need to do is add a few more pointers. Send your chest over your hands and draw your elbows toward each other as your arms straighten. Use the strength of your back muscles, leg muscles, and pelvic floor to lift up into Urdhva Dhanurasana. Gaze down at the floor between your hands. Stay for five breaths, then come down. Repeat up to two more times.

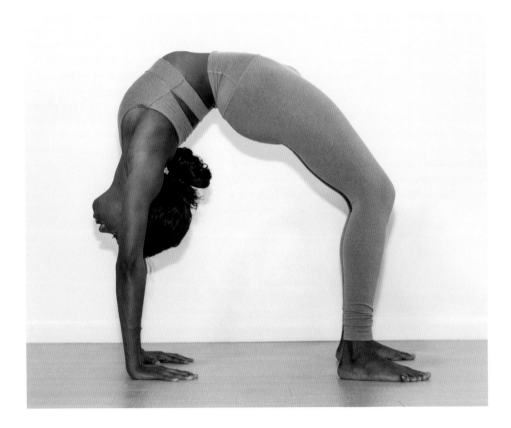

Warrior I

Virabhadrasana A

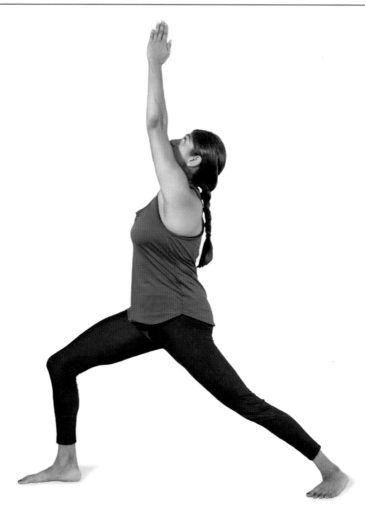

12

The mythology of *Virabhadrasana*, or Warrior Pose, tells the story of a warrior who fell to earth holding a sword above his head and landed in the shape of this pose. His name was Virabhadra, and he didn't start off peaceful. Created out of a lock of the Hindu deity Shiva's hair, Virabhadra was set on a mission of vengeance. But eventually he became a warrior for dharma, or goodness.

When we start the journey of yoga, we are not necessarily peaceful. We are often filled with petty ambitions, and we worship at the altar of power, money, and influence. But the practice works on our hearts and eventually we become humbler, until one day we too embrace the sword of dharma and become warriors of goodness in the world. Wherever you are on your journey, I hope this story inspires you to keep practicing.

◆◆◆◆◆◆ ◆ ◆◆◆◆◆◆

Start off in Samasthiti. Step your left foot back about three feet, gauging the distance according to your own height. Keep your legs straight and align your heels with each other. For those who are naturally flexible and have good balance, you might consider aligning your left arch with your right heel. Activate your pelvic floor and draw in your lower belly toward your spine.

Externally rotate your left hip joint to about forty-five degrees. Root down into the strength of your left leg and keep all your left toes on the ground. Slowly bend your right knee while drawing your right femur into its socket. Square your hips and chest forward. Avoid jutting your right knee forward and be sure that your right knee does not go beyond your right toes. Set up the foundation in your legs, and do not drop your hips below your knees. Eventually your right thigh will be

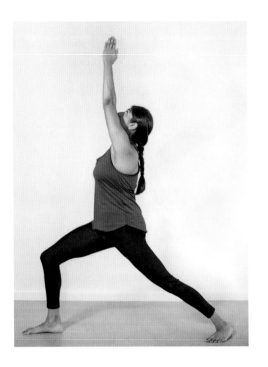

parallel with the ground. If your thighs start to burn, that is a good sign. Lift your ribs away from your hips and stack your torso along the centerline. Raise your arms into the centerline by externally rotating your shoulders, and gently press your palms together. Gaze toward your thumbs. Stay for five breaths, then return to Samasthiti. Repeat on the other side.

While Virabhadrasana A is typically entered from Downward-Facing Dog, it can be very difficult for many students to step forward and find the alignment. Instead, I'm presenting Warrior I in its most accessible entry. Once you become proficient here, you might try entering and exiting from Downward-Facing Dog.

Warrior I with a Wider Stance

Warrior I can be very challenging for larger bodies, pregnant women, or people with bad balance. Try widening your stance and take your legs wider. Imagine that there is a plank on your mat and align your feet on either side of the plank. Next, twist a little from beneath your rib cage to square your shoulders to the front of the mat. This variation makes trying to square your hips easier and may help you find better balance. If balance is an issue, try keeping one hand on the wall or a chair.

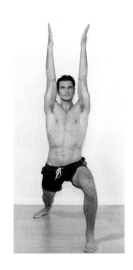

Warrior I with Arm Variations

Raising the arms is a challenging part of Warrior I. Tightness in the shoulders and preexisting neck issues often create obstacles to aligning the arms with the centerline. Try keeping your hands at your heart-center instead of raising your arms. Or if you are comfortable raising your arms but cannot gaze upward, try keeping your arms open and gaze forward. Line up your hands and shoulders and continue to work with the external rotation.

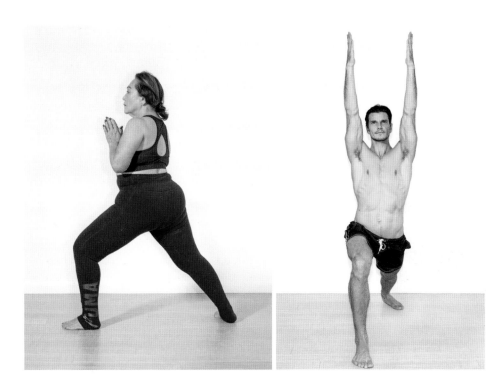

ALTERNATIVE TO WARRIOR I
Crescent Lunge Pose / Anjanayasana

Sometimes coming up into the full pose is simply not an option. Try *Anjanayasana*, or Crescent Lunge Pose, instead. When entering the pose, follow all the alignment pointers outlined above except those for your legs. Keep your hips parallel and rest your knee on the ground. Once you feel stable, work on lifting your knee and extending your leg. To transition into elevating your back knee, engage your pelvic floor, firm your quadriceps, and straighten your back leg while lifting your hips. If you are recovering from a knee injury or if your balance is challenged when you raise your arms above your head, this option will be extremely useful. Experiment with arm variations to find a comfortable position to practice.

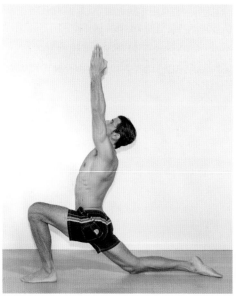
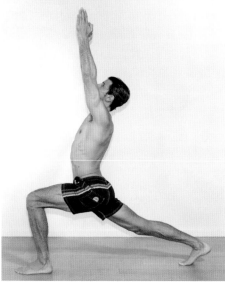

Standing Hand-to-Big-Toe Pose

Utthita Hasta Padangusthasana

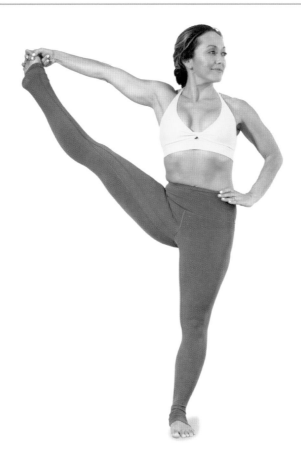

13

Balancing poses can be both challenging and humbling. You may feel like a failure or wonder if you're good enough. First, let yourself off the flexibility hook. Balancing poses are not stretching poses. You are here to work on your balance; remove from your mind anything that prevents you from working on the core lesson of the pose. So many students will attempt to stretch their hamstrings and hike their legs as high as possible. But that misses the point. *Utthita Hasta Padangusthasana*, or Standing Hand-to-Big-Toe Pose, is a balancing pose that articulates what flexibility you have. You must accept the limits of your flexibility to practice this asana well.

If you surpass your flexibility limits here, balance will be impossible. I advise you to err on the side of caution and underachievement with regards to the depth of flexibility, and put your effort into developing good balance.

The key to practicing balancing poses is all about the inner journey. By cultivating an inner state of faith and forgiveness, you will find the strength you need to pick yourself back up each time you fall. The truth is that the best way you learn how to balance is by falling. On a neuromuscular level, your body has to learn its own limits from direct experience. Your body's ability to sense where it is in space is called proprioception, and this function happens best through trial and error. In other words, you should not expect to be in balance for the first few hundred or even thousand attempts at a challenging pose. Instead, work with full faith that you will one day find balance and forgive yourself each time you stumble. Along the way to achieving the physical balance, you will learn mental and spiritual lessons that translate into your life.

✦✦✦✦✦✦ ◆ ✦✦✦✦✦✦

Utthita Hasta Padangusthasana is actually very advanced in its full expression. Instead of starting with the full pose, I am going to present the options first and then build up to the full expression. Advanced practitioners of many years still struggle with Utthita Hasta Padangusthasana, so I recommend that you go slowly and don't force yourself to do too much too soon. Instead, focus on the subtlety of the inner work and learn to meet and make peace with your body along the way.

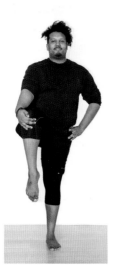

VARIATIONS

Standing Hand-to-Big-Toe Pose with a Bent Knee
Start off in Samasthiti. Activate your pelvic floor and draw in your lower belly. Root down into your left leg and shift your center of gravity slightly over your left foot. Throughout the pose, keep your left leg stable and strong. Avoid bending your left knee. Inhale as you bend your right knee, engage your core and thigh muscles, and draw in your right leg toward your chest. Align your right knee with your hip joint and keep your hip in parallel position. Use your hip flexion to sink the head of your right femur deeper into its socket. Wrap your right hand around your right shin and your left hand around the left side your waist. Gaze down toward the floor slightly forward. Stay for five breaths.

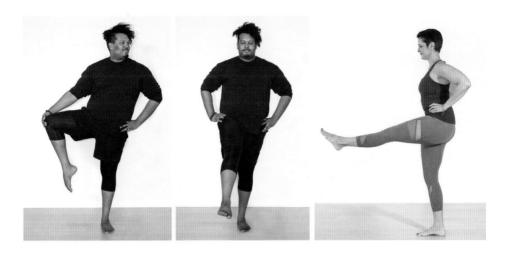

Next, bring extra attention to your right hip joint. Slowly, move your center of gravity even more toward the left as you roll through the external rotation of your right hip joint to bring your right knee gently out to the right side. Avoid hiking your right hip and keep your sitting bones as level as possible. Do not worry about how far to the side your right knee goes; instead, focus on the movement in your hip joint. Switch your gaze to the left. Stay for five breaths.

Shift your right leg back to parallel position and shift your center of gravity back slightly toward the center in a synchronous movement. Draw your right femur back into its socket and engage your abdominal muscles. Place both hands on your waist and straighten your right leg completely. It does not matter how high off the ground your right leg is. As long as it remains off the ground at least one inch, you are practicing the pose. If you lose your balance, just pick it back up and try again. Gaze toward your right toes. Stay for five breaths. Return to Samasthiti. Repeat on the left side.

Standing Hand-to-Big-Toe Pose with a Strap

Utthita Hasta Padangusthasana can be especially difficult for many students. If your legs are longer than your arms, or you have a bigger body, it may be difficult to hold your knee. Using a strap can make the pose more accessible. Straps lengthen your arms and help support the extension of your leg. The key to making successful use of the strap is to focus on the movement deep inside the hip joints. Do not use the strap to force your leg high or stretch your hamstrings.

Following the instructions outlined above, bend your left knee in toward your chest. Make a loop with the strap, hold the strap in your left hand and slide the

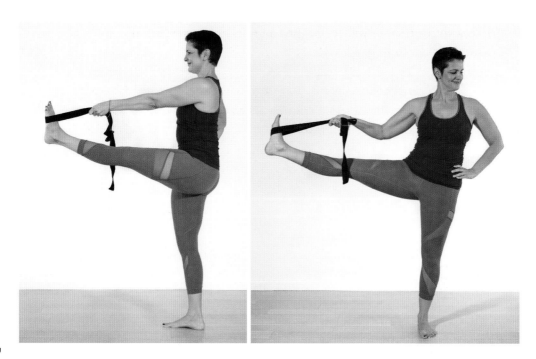

strap around the ball of your left foot. Bring your attention in toward your left hip joint, draw your femur into its socket, and extend your leg out in front of you. If you find that your leg only straightens when it is below the line of your hip joint, remove the strap and continue with the first option outlined above. If you find that your leg is comfortable at least in line with your hip joint, then proceed. You may also find that your leg wants to rise higher than your hip joint. Feel welcome to follow the natural extension of your hip, but do not force it or try to stretch your hamstring. Stay for five breaths, then follow the same method outlined above to bring your right leg out to the side, using external hip rotation. Finally, return to the center, remove your foot from the strap, place both hands at your waist, and lift your leg on its own for five breaths. Return to Samasthiti and repeat on the other side.

Standing Hand-to-Big-Toe Pose with a Chair or Wall

If you find balance to be exceedingly hard, then use a chair for extra support. If you are recovering from an illness, have vertigo, are a stroke victim, have flat feet, or just generally find balance challenging, using some additional support may make Utthita Hasta Padangusthasana more accessible.

To work with a chair or wall, place the hand that would rest on your waist on the chair or wall for support throughout the pose. If you need additional support, try placing your extended leg on a chair. Note that if you proceed with this option, you will need to come down and set up again in between all three variations of Utthita Hasta Padangusthasana. Do not be an overachiever. If using a wall or chair helps you find better balance and spatial orientation, practice with this assist until you feel more stable.

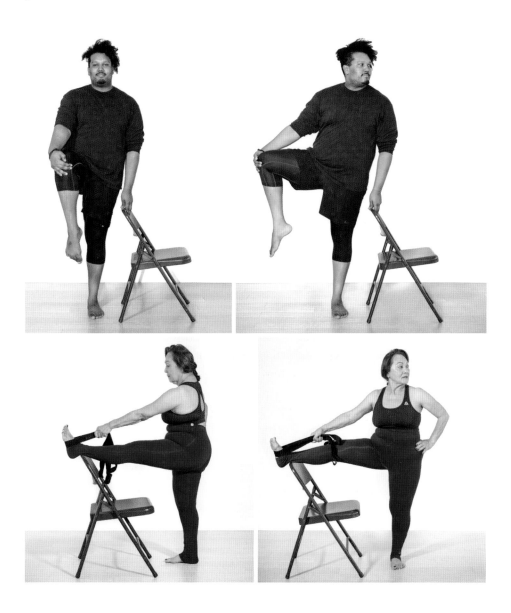

Standing Hand-to-Big-Toe Pose with Straight Legs

Remember that the full expression of Utthita Hasta Padangusthasana is quite advanced. You should be able to easily perform all the modifications before attempting this option. When you're ready, start off in Samasthiti. Activate your pelvic floor and draw in your lower belly. Root down into your right leg and shift your center of gravity slightly over your right foot. Throughout the pose, keep your right leg stable and strong. Avoid bending your right knee. Inhale as

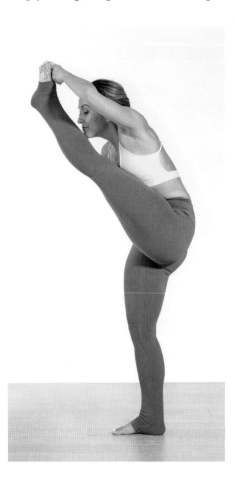

you bend your left knee, engage your core and thigh muscles, and draw in your left leg toward your chest. Align your left knee with your left hip joint and keep your left hip in parallel position.

Use your hip flexion to sink the head of your left femur deeper into its socket. Wrap your left index finger, middle finger, and thumb around your left big toe. Place your right hand on the right side of your waist. Gaze down toward the floor slightly forward. Bring your attention in toward your left hip joint, draw your femur into its socket and extend your leg out in front of you. Once your balance is established, send your pelvis back and fold your chest down toward your left knee. Stay for five breaths. Inhale, lift your torso, and return to standing balance. Next, bring extra attention to your left hip joint.

Slowly move your center of gravity even more toward the left as you roll through the external rotation of your right hip joint to bring your right leg gently out to the right side. Avoid hiking your right hip and keep your sitting bones as level as possible. Do not worry about how far to the side your right leg goes; instead, focus on the movement in your hip joint.

Switch your gaze to the left. Stay for five breaths. Then shift your leg back to parallel position and shift your center of gravity back slightly toward the center in a synchronous movement. Draw your right femur back into its socket and fold your chest down toward your right knee for one breath. Inhale, return to standing balance, place both hands on your waist, and straighten your right leg completely. Engage your abdominal muscles and firm your legs. It does not matter how high off the ground your right leg is, as long as it remains off the ground. Gaze toward your right toes. Stay for five breaths. Return to Samasthiti. Repeat on the left side.

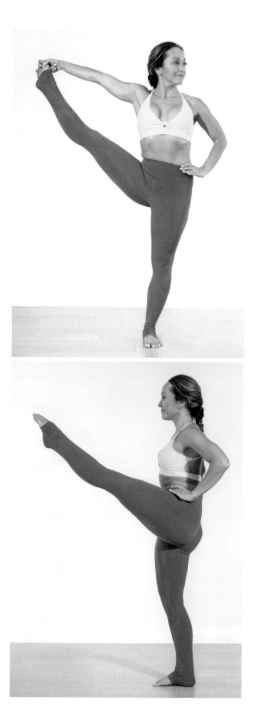

Tree Pose

Vrksasana

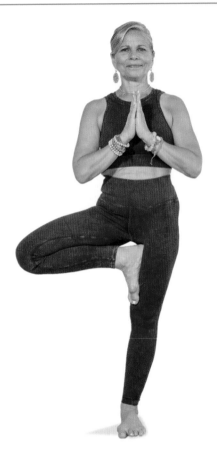

14

When you have the blessing of walking through a natural forest, you automatically appreciate the diversity of trees. The sheer variety of shapes, sizes, ages, and types makes it exhilarating to be in nature. We would never consider a tree unworthy because it didn't look like all the others—or if it was any less than the full expression of itself. If we can tune in to the beauty and uniqueness of each tree while we are hiking through a forest, we can use our yoga practice to tune in to that same beauty and uniqueness within ourselves. There is no better place to practice this mind-set than in *Vrksasana*, or Tree Pose.

◆◆◆◆◆◆ ◆ ◆◆◆◆◆◆

Start in Samasthiti. Activate your pelvic floor and draw in your lower belly. Root down into your left leg and shift your center of gravity slightly over your left foot. Throughout the pose, keep your left leg stable and strong. Avoid bending your left knee. Inhale as you bend your right knee slightly and come up onto the ball of your right foot. Keeping the ball of your right foot on the ground, externally rotate your right hip joint and gently angle your right foot and right knee out to the right. Do not worry how far out to the right you are able to angle your foot and knee. Simply explore the range of motion that your hip joint permits.

Place the heel of your right foot against your left ankle and press down into the floor through the ball of your foot to use your toes like a kickstand. Align your body along the central axis, engage your abdominal muscles, and think "up" along the spine. Inhale as you bring your hands to prayer position at the center of your chest. Gaze out to a single point, slightly forward and down. Stay for five breaths. Exhale and return to Samasthiti. Repeat on the other side.

If you feel comfortable here, you might be ready to try a more advanced Vrksasana. Inhale as you slide your right foot up along the inner edge of your left calf muscle. Fold the arch of your right foot along your left calf muscle; stabilize here by gently pressing your foot into your calf muscle. Firm your left leg and root down into the base of your left big toe, the base of your left little toe, and your left heel. Do not attempt to press your right foot into the inner edge of your knee or else you may apply undue pressure on your knee.

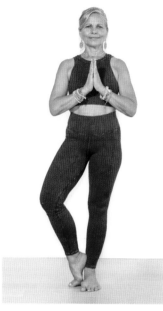

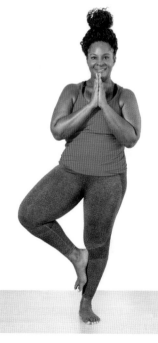

Tree Pose

77

Maintain your gaze at a single point, with hands in prayer position at the center of your chest. Stay for a few breaths here and determine whether you are ready to move on to a deeper version of Vrksasana. If so, slide your right foot up along the inner edge of your left thigh. Reach down with your hands and gently guide your right foot as close to your groin as possible. Once your right foot is in place, actively press into your left inner thigh. Activate your left inner thigh and press it gently toward your right foot. Hold your hands in prayer position at the center of your chest.

Finally, for a greater challenge to your balance, explore different hand positions. First, extend your arms out to the side and make a T shape. When holding the T-shape arms, extend your arms fully and spread your shoulder blades away from each other. Hold your shoulder joints in neutral position. Then, once you find your balance here, raise your hands above your head. Align your arms over your shoulders and externally rotate your shoulder joints. Fully straighten your arms. Maintain your gaze forward to a single point. Stay for five breaths. Then return to Samasthiti.

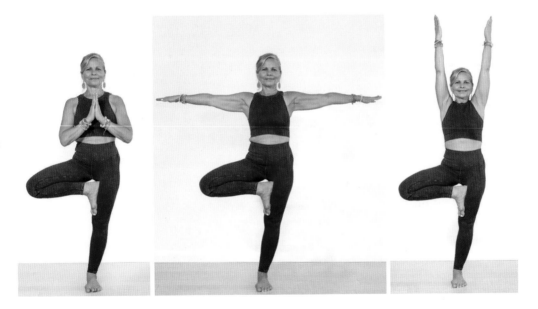

It's important to choose an option that works well for you. There is no competition in yoga practice. Think of all these variations of Vrksasana as naturally occurring trees in a forest. Choose which type of tree you'll be today and then be patient with yourself as you grow. Like a pine tree, you may spend fifteen to twenty years working on your root system before you sprout up.

Tree Pose with a Wall or a Chair

While these variations of Vrksasana are quite accessible, you may need some additional help with balancing. Standing near a wall or chair, but not touching it, can also help ground your sense of balance. When setting up for Vrksasana, stand with your straight leg closest to the wall or chair. Instead of bringing both hands to prayer position, bring one hand to the wall or place one hand on the back of the chair to support your balance. Don't worry about taking your hand off the wall or chair. Simply focus on your breath and feel your inner body. Much like new trees need a support system to plant their roots, you need ample time to build your foundation. You can move through all variations of Vrksasana with the assistance of a wall or chair.

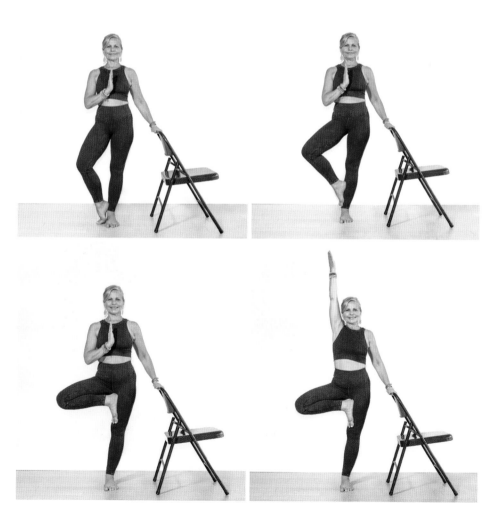

Standing Half Lotus / Ardha Baddha Padmottanasana

For students who find Vrksasana easy, try the much more advanced pose, *Ardha Baddha Padmottanasana*, or Standing Half Lotus. From the most advanced option outlined above, continue sliding your right foot along your left inner thigh until your right foot slides all the way up toward your hip crease into the position called Half Lotus. Do not force your knee. If you feel any pain in your knee while attempting this, return to Vrksasana. Guide your right foot into Half Lotus, snuggle the instep of your foot in toward your left hip crease, and allow your right knee to gently point down toward the ground. Hold your right foot with your left hand and slide your right hand around your back and reach toward your left elbow. Stay here for a few breaths.

Then, if your body gives you the green light to proceed, slide your right hand down toward your right foot and, if accessible, catch your right foot with your right hand. Allow your left hand to drape down by your side. Gaze out to a single point, slightly forward and down. Stay for five breaths. If you want to challenge your balance, try raising your left hand above your head. Finally, if your feet are comfortable, you might try folding forward from Standing Half Lotus.

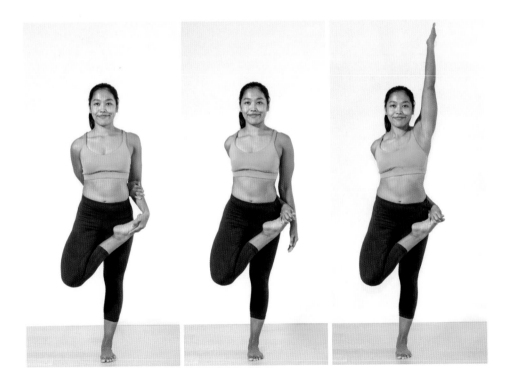

If you're ready to enter the full expression of the pose, then switch your gaze down to prepare. Exhale as you fold from your hip joint, place your left hand on the floor near your left foot, and drop your head close to your left shin. Gaze either down toward the floor or toward your nose. Stay for five breaths. Inhale and straighten your spine. Exhale there to stabilize and engage your pelvic floor. Inhale and come all the way up to standing. Exhale and return to Samasthiti. Repeat on the other side.

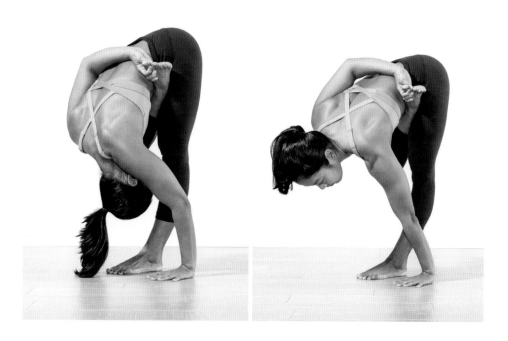

Pyramid Pose (Intense Side Stretch Pose)

Parsvottanasana

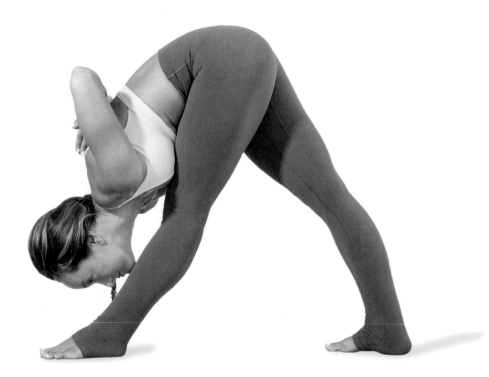

15

Standing forward folds make it easier to feel the deep inner work of your pelvic floor. Stabilizing your legs and allowing your torso to drape over your thighs encourages you to naturally draw in your lower belly. The key to entering forward folds is to place your attention on your inner body and let go of the need to force your body into a form. It's not about the size or shape of your body; the practice is an experience of subtlety in the space underneath your skin, in the region I refer to as the inner body. So, while most forward folds suggest that you draw inward and discover the empty space of your pelvis, this has nothing to do with the size of your lower belly. Instead, it's about developing aliveness in the network of muscles and flesh in the region underneath your navel and in the center of your pelvis.

Parsvottanasana is translated into English directly as Intense Side Stretch Pose, but most contemporary styles of yoga refer to it simply as Pyramid Pose. Start in Samasthiti. Activate your pelvic floor and draw in your lower abdominal muscles. Inhale as you step out to the right about three feet. Turn your hips toward the back of your mat and turn your right hip joint outward at forty-five degrees. There are three possible alignments for your feet. If your balance in challenged, leave an inch or more between your heels. If you have good balance and medium flexibility, align your heels with each other. If you have both good balance and flexibility, then align your left heel with your right arch.

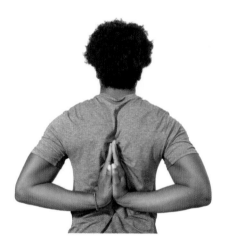 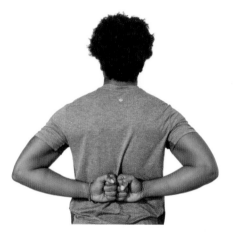

Place your hands in prayer position behind your back or grab your elbows. Facilitate an internal rotation of your shoulder joints by dropping the head of your humerus forward. Keep your collarbone broad and avoid collapsing your chest. Exhale as you fold forward. Initiate the movement of folding forward from behind your pubic bone, in your hip joints. Think of your torso as one unit and send your sitting bones back and up as your chest reaches down toward your right knee.

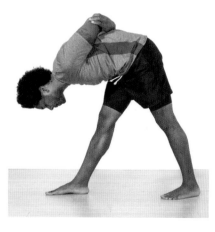

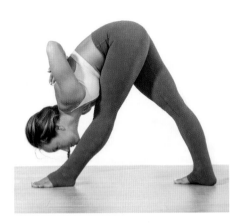

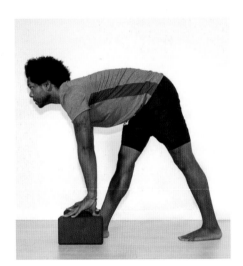

Yet, at the same time, relax the muscles of your back so that you have a sense of ease along your spine.

If your back muscles are overly active, you will prevent yourself from deeply folding forward. In order to keep your hips relatively level throughout *Parsvottanasana*—Intense Side Stretch Pose or Pyramid Pose—you will need to feel as though you send a bit more weight into the forward leg. Gaze toward the toes of your forward leg. Stay for five breaths, then repeat on the other side.

VARIATION
Pyramid Pose with Blocks

Sometimes the pressure on your forward leg in Parsvottanasana is just too much for your hamstring to handle. Sometimes even modifying by holding your elbows is too intense for your shoulders. Try using blocks at both sides of your extended foot to ground your arms. This modification will help you find a better foundation in your legs. Follow the instructions outlined above, except you now have the option of placing your hands on blocks. As you fold forward, place your fingertips or your whole palms flat on the blocks. If you are unable to comfortably reach the blocks, try placing your hands on the wall. Gaze toward your right toes. Stay for five breaths, then repeat on the other side.

Seated Forward Fold

Paschimattanasana

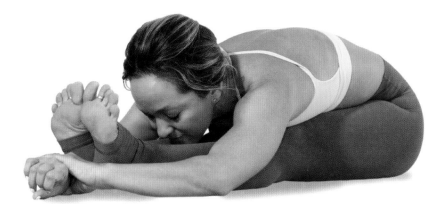

16

Seated forward folds are an essential part of every yoga practice—and they're not easy. I still remember the first time that I tried to fold forward. My back was rounded, and I could not touch my toes. I had no idea what it meant to pivot from the hips, nor how to access my pelvic floor. I thought my arms were just too short to reach my feet. But with practice and good technique, my body opened. And yours will too. Don't be discouraged if it feels difficult or confronting at first. The work of yoga is to rise up and meet the challenge with a heart full of expectant faith and joy.

Paschimattanasana is often simply referred to as Seated Forward Fold but is translated directly into English as Intense Westward Stretch. As you begin your practice of Paschimattanasana, you will experience some of the deep cleansing work that is the essence of the practice. All forward folds cleanse the digestive system and optimize organ function. The result is often more energy and better assimilation of nutrients.

With this pose, it is very important for you to be aware of your inner commentary. Many students come to yoga practice and assume that you have to be very thin in order to fold forward or benefit from the practice. That is patently untrue. All sizes and shapes can bend forward and receive the deep benefits of the practice.

If you start thinking negative thoughts about the size or shape of your body as you fold forward, note your self-judgments and see if you can reframe your thoughts to celebrate the fact that you are practicing. Plant the seeds of loving thoughts about your body as you practice.

✦✦✦✦✦ ◆ ✦✦✦✦✦

Start off in the seated staff pose called *Dandasana*, which is used as a preparatory pose for many seated poses. Sit on the floor and straighten your legs. Activate your pelvic floor, draw in your lower abdominal muscles, and float your rib cage away from your hips. Firm your quadriceps, press the bases of your big toes together, and allow a gentle internal rotation of your hip joints. Keep your shoulders and neck relaxed. Pivot forward from your hip joints, send your sitting bones back, and fold into your hip creases.

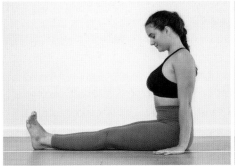
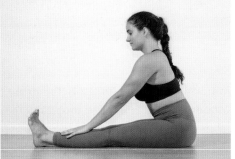

Extend your arms and wrap your index fingers, middle fingers, and thumbs around your big toes. If you cannot reach your big toes, either wrap your fingers around your shinbones or use a strap around the balls of your feet. Use whichever

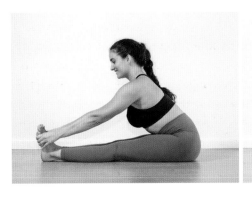
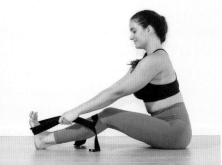

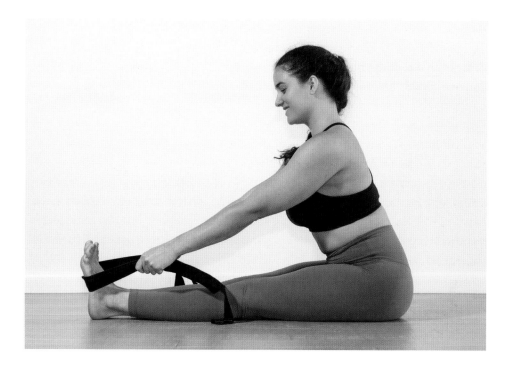

grip feels most comfortable and allows you to keep your legs straight. Avoid bending your knees in Paschimattanasana unless you have a hamstring or back injury and are modifying to protect your preexisting condition. If you simply feel tight, then choose an arm position that allows you to work with straight legs. The hamstrings only effectively release when the quadriceps engage and the legs are straight. Bending your knees to avoid discomfort in the center of the hamstring muscles unfortunately prevents the stretching that is exactly what Paschimattanasana targets.

Once you establish a comfortable grip, inhale to create space between the joints of your spine. Exhale as you draw back your femurs and fold forward from your hips. Relax your back muscles but avoid overly rounding your back. While it may feel very difficult to keep the muscles of your lower belly drawn in, try anyway. The action of sucking in and elongating your abdominal muscles supports your lumbar spine in the action of forward bending. Draw in your lower ribs slightly as your chest reaches forward, out and over your thighs. If your head does not touch your shins, gaze forward to your toes. If your chin touches your shins, gaze forward to your toes. If your forehead touches your knees, gaze toward your nose. Stay for five breaths. Then return to Dandasana.

VARIATIONS

Seated Forward Fold on a Blanket

One of the most difficult aspects of Seated Forward Fold is finding the pivot in your hip joints. If you spend most of your days sitting in a chair, then it is highly likely that your hips do not naturally pivot. Similarly, if you are a runner or just have a lot of tightness around your lower back,

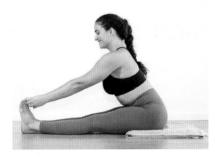

your hamstrings may be extra tight. In this case, it's advised to sit on a blanket when entering Paschimattanasana. Elevating your hips even slightly encourages a deeper forward fold originating from your hip joints. Once your sitting bones are lifted off the ground, it may also be easier to get the feeling that they reach back as you fold forward. Finally, elevating your hips helps release some of the pressure on your lower back that can sometimes be an obstacle in forward folds. To use a blanket, fold up a yoga blanket to provide an inch or less height. Then sit in approximately the middle of the folded blanket and follow the instructions outlined above.

Seated Forward Fold with Wider Legs

Bigger bodies may find the traditional alignment very challenging. Depending on the size and shape of your thighs, it may or may not be possible to press the bases of your big toes into each other. Similarly, the size and shape of your lower belly may inhibit forward folding. If you notice either of these obstacles when practicing Paschimattanasana, try bringing your feet just a little apart. Align your heels with your hip joints to place your feet hip-width apart. Consider using a block between your feet so that the inner edges of your feet can still press together. Follow the instructions outlined above and remember to adjust your hand grip according to your level of flexibility.

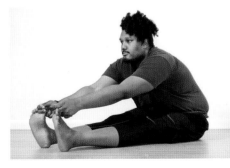
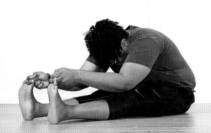

Head-to-Knee Pose

Janu Sirsasana A

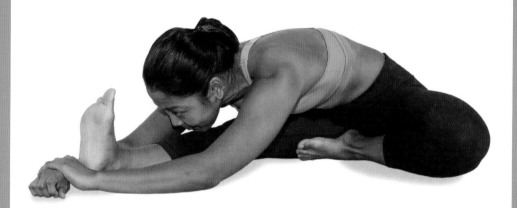

17

The difficult and challenging poses in yoga garner the most attention, but the healing aspects of practice often happen in the basic postures. *Janu Sirsasana* A, or Head-to-Knee Pose, is a basic forward fold that begins to unlock the depth of hip rotation. The inner work available in this pose has the power to reset and stabilize the sacrum and relieve lower back pain. The action of forward folding encourages the inner cleansing work that begins in Paschimattanasana. Remember not to force yourself into a deeper physical form. Instead, focus on deepening your breath and diving into the inner experience.

✦ ✦ ✦ ✦ ✦ ◆ ✦ ✦ ✦ ✦ ✦

Start off in Dandasana. Activate your pelvic floor, draw in your lower abdominal muscles and float your rib cage away from your hips. Bend your right knee in toward your chest and slide your right foot up as close to the back of your right thigh as possible. Drop your right knee out to the side and rotate your right hip joint externally. Draw your right heel in as close to your pubic bone as possible.

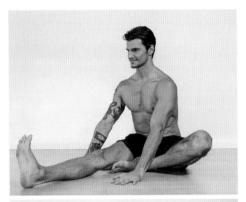

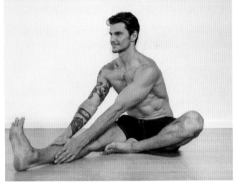

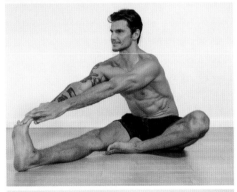

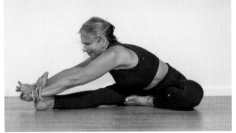

Firm your left quadriceps and gently internally rotate your left hip joint. Keep your right knee out to the side approximately ninety degrees from your pubic bone. Orient the center of your chest toward your left knee. Keep your shoulders and neck relaxed. Pivot forward from your hip joints, send back your sitting bones, and fold into your left hip crease. Extend your arms and find a comfortable place to rest your hands on the ground. This may be the limit of your flexibility for today. If so, respect that and avoid forcing yourself to go deeper if your body is not ready.

Explore different hand positions that allow you to work without compromising the integrity of your breath and the alignment of the pose. Try wrapping your hands around your shin or extending your arms to lightly grip your foot or toes. You may find that your hands wrap around your left foot completely. Whether you bind your wrist, hold on to the outer edges of your left foot, use a strap, or rest your hands on your left shinbone, find the position that works best for your body. Keep your left leg straight and ground down into your left heel. Avoid bending your left knee unless you have a preexisting injury that you are working to rehabilitate.

Once you establish a comfortable grip, inhale to create space between the joints of your spine. Exhale as you draw back your left femur and fold forward from your hips. Relax your back muscles but avoid overly rounding your back. While it may feel very difficult to keep your lower belly muscles drawn in, try anyway. The action of sucking in and elongating your abdominal muscles

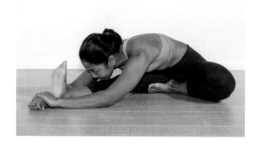

supports the lumbar spine in the action of forward bending. Draw your lower ribs slightly in as your chest reaches toward your left shin. Ideally your chest is center to your left knee. While you fold forward, keep the area between your right calf muscle and thigh knit together. Avoid separating these two areas and keep your knee sealed.

As you fold forward, send back your sitting bones and allow your right leg to roll slightly forward (but note that your hip is still externally rotated). If your head does not touch your shin, gaze forward toward your toes. If your chin touches your shin, gaze forward toward your toes. If your forehead touches your knees, then gaze toward your nose. Stay for five breaths. Then return to Dandasana and repeat on the other side.

VARIATIONS

Head-to-Knee Pose on a Blanket and with a Strap

If folding forward is difficult and you used a blanket when entering Paschimattanasana, you might also try elevating your hips here. Even a slight elevation encourages a deeper forward fold originating from your hip joints. Once your sitting bones are lifted off the ground, it may also be easier to get the feeling that they reach back as you fold forward. Finally, elevating your hips helps release some of the pressure on your lower back that can sometimes be an obstacle in forward folds.

To use a blanket, fold up a yoga blanket to provide an inch or less height. Then sit in approximately the middle of the folded blanket and follow the instructions outlined above.

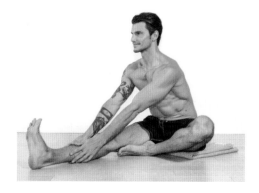

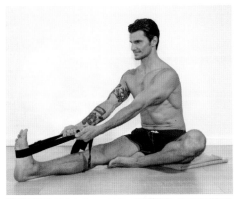

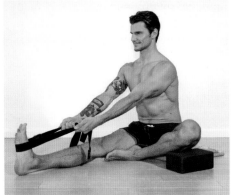

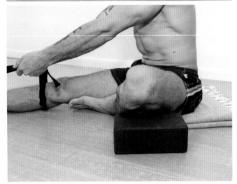

If none of the hand positions outlined above work, then use a strap around the ball of your left foot.

Head-to-Knee Pose with a Block

External rotation of the hip joint and deep hip flexion can be quite difficult for some students. If you are unable to close your knee joint fully, you may find the leg position inaccessible. To make the pose more accessible, try using a block under your right knee. Place the block directly under your bent knee to provide support, but do not let the block lift your knee higher than it would naturally fall. If you have a knee injury or you feel pressure or pain on the outer edge of your right knee, use a block or another support under your right knee to provide a firm foundation. Never push through knee pain in your yoga practice.

Marichi's Pose A

Marichasana A

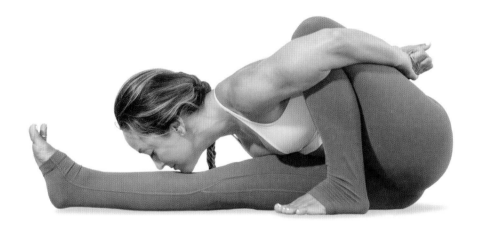

18

Seated poses encourage a subtle turning inward of the mind and cultivate a meditative state. *Marichasana* A, or Pose Dedicated to the Sage Marichi, is a therapeutic and cleansing pose that can easily be made accessible for all. The name *Marichi* means "ray of light," and this ancient sage is known as one of the seven great sages whose virtues are extolled in the Vedas. Regular practice of Marichasana A, and other supporting poses, can relieve chronic lower back pain. As you move into Marichasana A, place extra emphasis on your breath and inner experience. Do not force or rush through to some physical goal. Instead, keep your mind steadily attentive to the subtlety of the inner realms. And, of course, breathe deeply.

◆ ◆ ◆ ◆ ◆ ◆ ◆ ◆ ◆ ◆ ◆ ◆ ◆

Start off in Dandasana. Activate your pelvic floor and draw in your lower abdominal muscles. Bend your right knee and bring your right heel as close to the back of your right thigh as possible. Ideally align your right foot with your right sitting bone. Root down into the base of your right big toe, little toe, and heel. Keep your left leg straight and root down into your left heel. Track your right knee in line with your right ankle and allow your right ankle to move into flexion as you

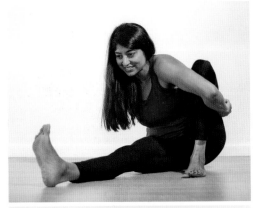

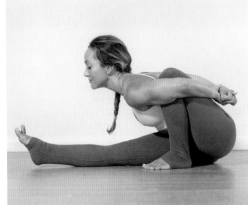

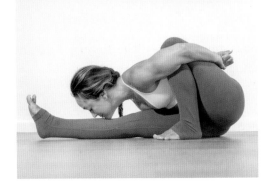

pivot slightly forward. Engage your left quadriceps and stabilize your left leg. Slide your torso forward and around your right thigh. Extend your right arm and drop your right shoulder as far down around your right shin as possible. Internally rotate your right shoulder and bend your right elbow around your right shin. Lift up your fingers around the outer edge of your right thigh and place the outer edge of the palm along the right side of your lower back. Drop your chest and allow your sitting bones to elevate slightly, but keep them grounded by firmly activating your pelvic floor.

Internally rotate your left shoulder and gently wrap your left hand around your back. Interlace the fingers of your hands together or wrap your right fingers around your left wrist. Avoid twisting your chest to the left to go deeper or force your hands to bind. Instead, focus on internally rotating both shoulders and dropping your chest down. Exhale as you fold your chest forward, aligning the center of your chest to your left knee. Maintain a slight internal rotation in your left leg to encourage a deeper forward fold. As much as you fold forward with your chest toward your left knee, pull with equal force back and down with your right hip. Avoid dumping weight toward the left. Gaze toward your left toes. Stay for five breaths and return to Dandasana. Repeat on the other side.

Marichasana A with a Strap and a Blanket

Marichasana A can be difficult for bigger bodies and tighter shoulders. Rather than struggling to fit the mold, modify the pose so that it works for your body. Place a blanket under your hips or sit on a bolster, cushion, or block and extend your legs to Dandasana. For this option, leave more than a hand's distance between your right foot and your left inner thigh. The slightly wider positioning of your right foot makes the bind more accessible and helps keep your right hip joint from externally rotating.

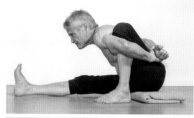

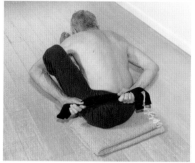

Follow all the alignment pointers and technical instructions outlined above. If you are not able to reach your hands together, grab a strap or towel with your left hand as you reach around your back. Avoid twisting your chest to the left to go deeper. Instead, focus on internally rotating both shoulders and dropping your chest down. Exhale as you fold your chest forward, aligning the center of your chest to your left knee. Maintain a slight internal rotation in your left leg to encourage a deeper forward fold. Avoid dumping weight toward the left. Gaze toward your left toes. Stay for five breaths and return to Dandasana. Repeat on the other side.

Marichasana A Hugging the Knee

Sometimes attempting any variation of the bind is simply inaccessible. Bigger bodies may find that there is simply not enough space to drop the torso around the thigh. Or students who cannot bend their knees more than ninety degrees due to injuries or knee-replacement surgeries may not get the angle required to modify the bind. In order to make Marichasana A accessible, try letting go of the need to bind at all. Instead, wrap your right hand around your thigh, hold your shin from the outside, and draw back your right thigh. Place your left hand on the floor for support and lean slightly forward and toward the left. Stay here for five breaths. Experiment with sitting on the floor and sitting on a blanket to see which is more comfortable.

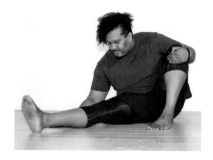

Marichi's Pose C

Marichasana C

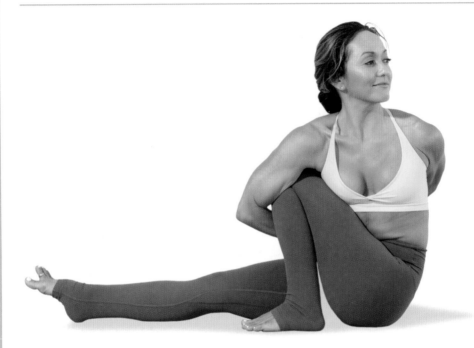

19

There are many poses named after the sage Marichi. In some ways, he was considered a progenitor of humankind who is known most by his descendants. It is no surprise that we include at least two of the prolific variations of Marichasana in this yoga journey. A sister pose to Marichasana A, Marichasana C twists the spine. Twisting, a crucial lesson in the yoga journey, cleanses the digestive system and all organs of the abdomen. Since breathing can be challenging while entering deep twists, the inner work of Marichasana C often revolves around finding comfort amid discomfort. Eventually, over many years of practice, it is possible to maintain a deep and fluid breath while in Marichasana C.

So many students wrongly associate the size and shape of their bodies with success along the yoga journey. I've heard many students tell me that they simply would never be able to twist because of the size of their torso or belly. Most get discouraged when they look at their size compared to the mainstream image of yoga.

But I'm here to tell you that size and shape are not requirements to practice, nor are they statements of worthiness or even health. As a yoga teacher for over twenty years, I have seen all different sizes and shapes successfully practice this asana and many others. I've also seen very thin, apparently healthy bodies with six-pack abs unable to twist, fold, or bend. If there is one thing that I'd like this pose to teach you, it's that thin and healthy are not the same. You can be razor thin and unhealthy, and you can be curvy and healthy. Place your attention on health, nourishment, and self-love.

◆ ◆ ◆ ◆ ◆ ◆ ◆ ◆ ◆ ◆ ◆ ◆ ◆

Start off in Dandasana. Activate your pelvic floor and draw in your lower abdominal muscles. Bend your right knee and bring your right heel as close to the back of your right thigh as possible. Ideally align your right foot with your right sitting bone. Root down into the base of your right big toe, little toe, and heel. Keep your left leg straight and root down into your left heel. Track your right knee in line with your right ankle and allow your right ankle to move into flexion as you pivot slightly forward. Engage your left quadriceps and stabilize your left leg. Ground the head of your right femur deeper into its socket. Start to angle your torso over to the right side by moving laterally. Aim the center of your chest around the outer edge of your right knee. Once the lateral stretch is established, gently pivot your spine around its axis and twist from each joint of your spine. Naturally most of the twisting action is centered around your thoracic spine and rib cage. Keep your chest and collarbone open and broad. Avoid dumping weight into the back of your spine. Reach your left arm around the outer edge of your right thigh. Once your left elbow passes the plane of your shinbone, internally rotate your left shoulder and wrap your left elbow around your right shin. Keep your left shoulder dropping down and around your right leg. Place your left fingers around your left hip crease. Exhale as you reach your right arm around your back and interlace your fingers together or hold your left wrist with your right fingers. Keep both sitting bones firmly planted on the ground. Avoid too much internal rotation of your right hip joint and keep your right knee in line with your right hip. Gaze to the right. Stay for five breaths. Return to Dandasana and repeat on the other side.

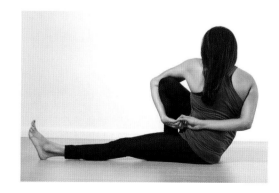

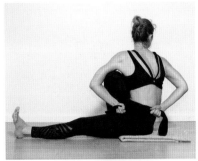

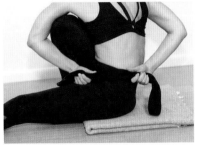

Marichasana C with a Strap and a Blanket

To make the pose more accessible, place a blanket under your hips or sit on a bolster, cushion, or block and extend your legs to Dandasana. For this option, leave more than a hand's distance between your right foot and your left inner thigh. The slightly wider positioning of your right foot makes the bind more accessible and helps keep your right hip joint from externally rotating. Follow all the alignment pointers and technical instructions outlined above. If you are not able to reach your hands together, then use a strap or towel. Place a strap or towel on your left hip crease before you start. Instead of binding your hands together, gently hold the strap and walk your hands closer together.

Marichasana C, No Bind with a Block

If twisting or binding is difficult, try one of these no-bind modifications. Following the instructions outlined above, instead of bending your left elbow around your right shinbone, keep your left arm straight. Rest your fingers on the ground or a block. Instead of reaching your right arm around your back, rest your right fingertips on the ground and gently push your weight forward.

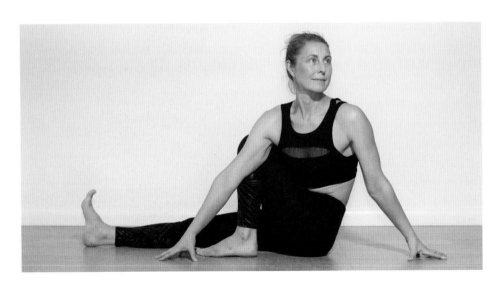

Or if reaching your left arm around your right leg is too difficult, snuggle your left elbow in front of your right shin, hug your right leg in toward your body, and gently pivot around your spinal axis toward the left.

Marichasana C Hugging the Knee

Sometimes attempting any variation of the bind is simply inaccessible. Bigger bodies may find that there is simply not enough space to wrap the torso around the thigh. Or students who cannot bend their knees more than ninety degrees due to injuries or knee-replacement surgeries may not get the angle required to modify the bind. Similarly, shoulder injuries may make the bind ill-advised. In order to make Marichasana C accessible, try letting go of the need to bind at all. Instead, wrap your left arm around your right shin, hold your upper right thigh from the outside, and draw your right knee forward to encourage a gentle internal rotation of your right hip joint. Avoid hiking your right hip off the ground, and engage your pelvic floor to keep your hips grounded. Place your right hand on the floor behind your hips for support and actively push your weight forward. Avoid leaning back or dumping weight into your lower back. Create as much length and space in your spine as possible and twist to the right. Keep your right knee as close to your chest as possible and look to the right. Stay here for five breaths. Experiment with sitting on the floor and sitting on a blanket to see which is more comfortable.

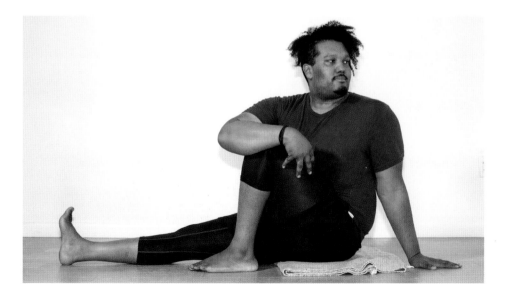

Boat Pose

Navasana

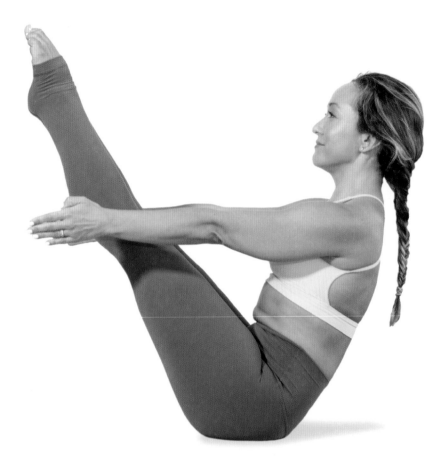

20

Regular yoga practice encourages a strong and healthy core. However, do not equate a strong core with a thin abdomen. The two do not necessarily go hand in hand. Instead of worrying about the size of your torso when practicing *Navasana*, or Boat Pose, direct your attention to the subtle work of your pelvic floor. Let the bowl of your pelvis be like the hull of a boat and balance the weight of your body with ease.

Start off in Dandasana. Activate your pelvic floor and draw in your lower abdominal muscles toward your spine. Bend your knees at an angle of ninety degrees or less to encourage a gentle hip flexion. Adduct your thighs to keep your knees together. Root down into the space between your sitting bones and your tailbone. Firm the muscles of your abdominal wall and consciously draw in toward the centerline of your torso with the transverse abdominals and internal obliques. Wrap your hands around your upper shins, just below the knees. Slowly extend and straighten your arms. Check to see if you feel stable. If not, then simply remain here. If so, point your feet and roll up to the tips of your toes. If you feel stable, you may be able to progress further into Navasana. Shift a little of your weight back, engage your entire abdominal cavity by drawing inward, and draw in your thighs toward your chest to lift your feet off the ground. Balance here with your arms extended. If you feel stable, straighten your legs. Straightening your legs in Navasana is a very advanced movement that requires a good deal of practice, strength, and flexibility. Don't force it. Work to the edge of a comfortable discomfort but don't push beyond a reasonable limit. Gaze toward your toes. Stay for five breaths, then return to Dandasana.

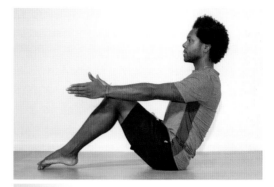
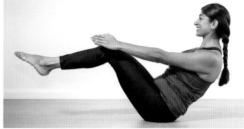
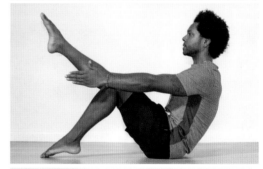
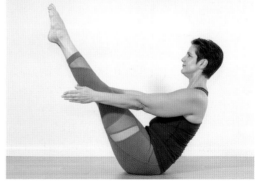

Boat Pose with Knees Slightly Apart

If you find it painful or inaccessible to keep your knees both together and close to the chest, take your knees farther apart to enter Navasana. If possible, keep your toes together. Make sure you are not rolling past your sitting bones. Lengthen your spine upward by rooting into your sitting bones as you broaden and expand your chest. Use the muscles of your abdomen to build a strong front body without rounding your back. Follow the same stages outlined above while keeping your knees slightly apart.

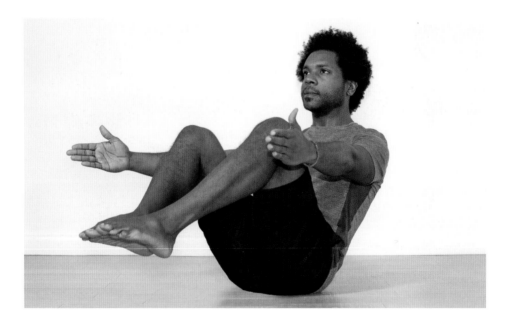

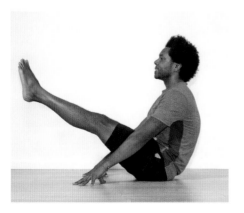

Boat Pose with Hand Support

If straightening your legs causes back pain or dumps weight into your lower back, try using your hands for support. Instead of straightening your arms at the beginning of the pose, leave your hands on the floor to support your spine. Then, when entering the full expression of Navasana, gently wrap your hands around the outer edges of your calf muscles. Use the grip to lightly ease the burden of the pose, but keep careful attention on activating your core.

Boat Pose with Support

If all the modifications listed so far are still too difficult, place your feet against the wall or on blocks to enter Navasana. Press the soles of your feet firmly into the wall as you lean your torso back into the strength of your core, stopping once you feel your core muscles engage.

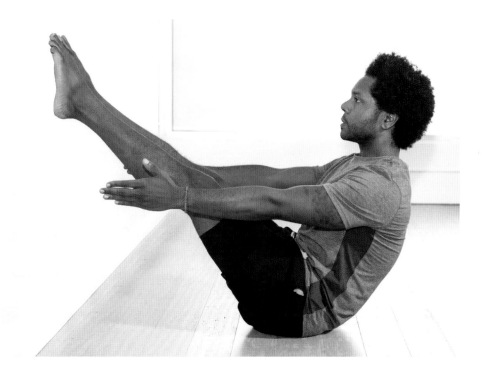

Reverse Plank
Purvattanasana

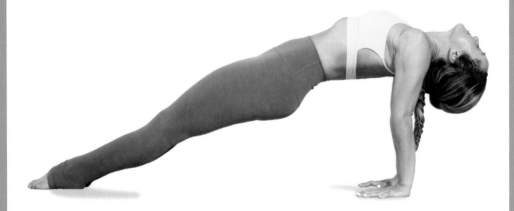

21

Understanding the basics of movement mechanics is key to awakening your inner body. Once your mind and body are in unity, a deep sense of peace pervades. Along the way there are poses that will be easy and others that will be a struggle. *Purvattanasana*, known most commonly as Reverse Plank, is directly translated into English as "Intense Eastward Stretch." This pose will most likely be more of a struggle than a feeling of ease at first. I've been practicing for over twenty years and I still find this lift-up quite difficult. So don't be surprised if you find it challenging as well. Taken together with Paschimattanasana and Dandasana, this trio represents the three basic positions of the spine: flexion, neutral, and extension. Putting in the work here opens the door to deeper backbends.

◆ ◆ ◆ ◆ ◆ ◆ ◆ ◆ ◆ ◆ ◆ ◆ ◆

Start off in Dandasana. Activate your pelvic floor and draw in the muscles of your lower abdomen toward your spine and elongate the abdomen. This may seem counterintuitive, but be careful not to engage or tighten your lower abs, or pooch the lower abdominal muscles outward. Instead, find a new way to recruit the muscles of the lower abdomen by drawing them both inward and upward.

Press the bases of your big toes in toward each other, point your feet, and internally rotate your hip joints. Note that the internal rotation of your hip joints is different than merely adducting your thighs. The action of squeezing your legs together may or may not internally rotate your hip joints, so be conscious of your muscular activation. Remember that it's better to do less correctly than just hit it hard and miss the subtlety of the inner work.

Keeping your hips in place, reach your hands back behind your pelvis and roll back onto your sacrum. Place the heels of your hands on the ground, point your fingers toward your pelvis, and internally rotate your shoulders. Inhale as you lift your chest to its maximum distance away from your hips. Exhale. Inhale and expand your chest and send your hips up and forward to lift up. Avoid clenching your gluteal muscles. Instead, use the muscles of your pelvic floor to support your hips from underneath. Be sure that your neck feels supported. Gently drop your head back to rest on your trapezius muscles and gaze toward your nose. Stay for five breaths. Then come down and return to Dandasana. You may find it challenging to breathe. If so, go slowly.

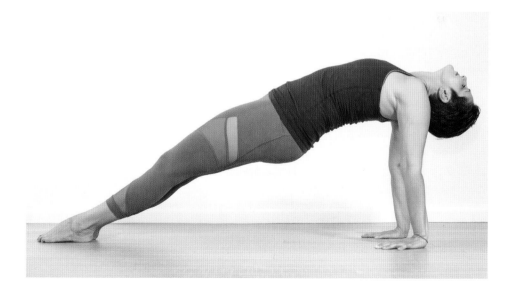

VARIATIONS

Reverse Plank with Bent Knees and a Block

It can be very difficult to lift the full weight of your body in Purvattanasana. Try a modified tabletop position instead. Following the instructions outlined above, start off with your knees slightly bent. Instead of straightening your legs, keep your knees bent and your feet hip-width apart. As you inhale and lift your hips up and forward, your knees will form a ninety-degree angle. If you have a hard time activating your legs, try holding a block between your knees. Placing a block between your knees helps keep your knees tracking in line with your hips and encourages just enough internal rotation to free the sacrum. Stay for five breaths here, then return to Dandasana.

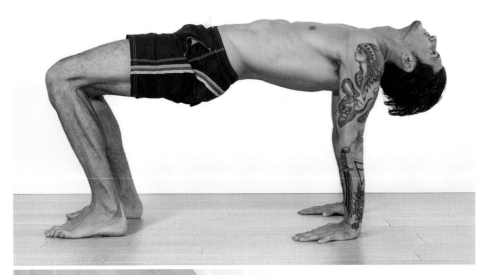

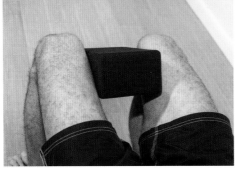

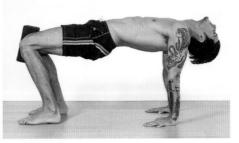

Half Reverse Plank

If you have a wrist or shoulder injury, it is not advised for you to bear weight on your arms. Instead of lifting up fully into Purvattanasana, stay in the preparatory pose where your chest is lifted. Do not lift your hips. Stay for five breaths here, then return to Dandasana.

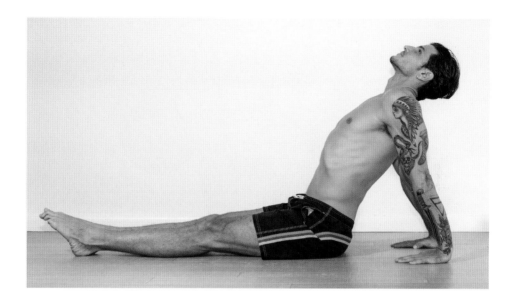

Camel Pose

Ustrasana

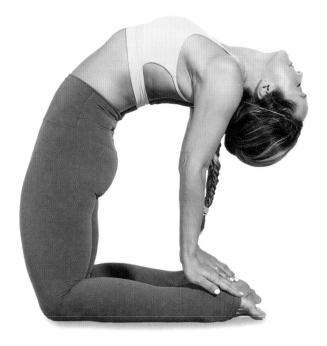

22

Backbending is such an important part of yoga practice. Moving deeply into your spine increases energy and stimulates so many vital body functions. Creating space between the joints of your spine also often relieves lower back pain. Since the main epicenter of backbending happens deep within the joints of your spine, your nervous system is also stimulated and cleansed. This can mean that the journey into backbends is sometimes also a journey into emotions. No matter what feelings arise, all that matters is that you cultivate an attitude of feeling and awareness. You do not need to solve any problems or go through a therapy session. All you have to do is feel whatever arises as it arises. Since backbending can be intense, it's important that your body is safe. You should never feel any sharp pinching sensations in the joints of your spine or any joint throughout your body. If you feel any sharp pinching sensations, calmly come out of the pose.

Ustrasana, or Camel Pose, is a relatively accessible backbend that will teach you the basics of spinal extension. Start off in kneeling position. Place your thighs about hip-width apart. Engage your pelvic floor and draw in your lower abdominal muscles toward your spine. Gently coax your hip joints into a subtle internal rotation. Point your feet and root down through your knees, shins, and feet. Inhale as you lift your ribs away from your hips. Place your hands in prayer position and create as much space as possible between the joints of your spine. Do not drop your head back. Stay here if you feel challenged. If you are ready to progress, dangle your arms by your sides and interlock your fingers behind your sacrum. Internally rotate your shoulders, lift up the center of your chest and start to engage the muscles of your back. Find the neck position that feels most supported, ideally not tucked in or dropped entirely back. Stay for a few breaths. Do not progress further if you feel challenged. Finally, to enter the full expression of Ustrasana, release your hands and reach the heels of your hands back toward the heels of your feet. Point your fingers in the same direction as your toes. Once you make contact, actively press down into your feet with your hands, rotate your shoulders internally, and drop your head back. Gaze toward your nose. Maintain as much length and space between the joints of your spine as possible. Stay for five breaths. When you are ready to come up, send your hips forward, then lift your rib cage onto the foundation of your pelvis and lastly bring up your head. Rest in Child's Pose.

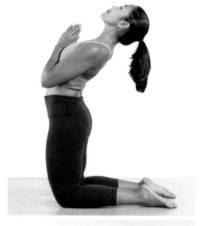

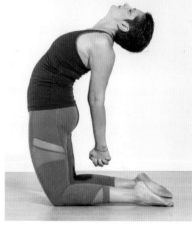

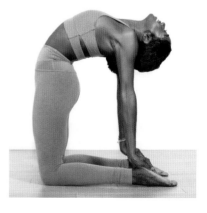

Camel Pose with Blocks

Elevate your heels by curling your toes under. Place a block beside each heel on the highest height setting. Place your hands on your hips and lift your ribs away from your hips. Following the instructions outlined above, reach your hands back to the blocks positioned on either side of your feet.

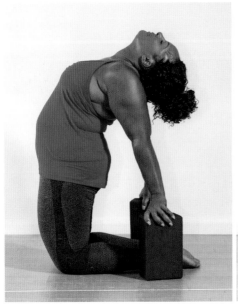
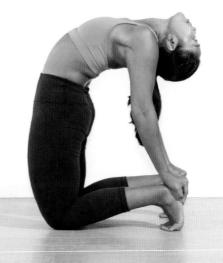

Pigeon Pose
Nidra Kapotasana

23

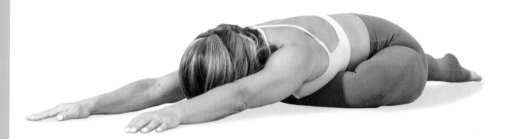

Many people have a love-hate relationship with Pigeon Pose. It's a great hip opener with several relaxing and rejuvenating benefits. But it is also really challenging. Since this is a pose that is recommended to hold for longer than the traditional five breaths, there is an opportunity for you to deepen your inner awareness. Sometimes emotions tend to bubble up to the surface in Pigeon Pose. The hips are widely understood to be storehouses of old emotions, particularly unprocessed feelings of trauma. If something deep arises during your practice, don't be disturbed. Remain calm and equanimous. Focus on the breath. Tune in to the sensations without judging or trying to solve them. Practice being present with your pain.

Pigeon, the English name for this pose, is derived from *Eka Pada Raja Kapotasana*, an advanced yoga pose. The leg position in this difficult asana is the foundation for the restorative pose most yoga schools simply refer to as Pigeon. However, it should be noted that there is in fact another pose that is officially called Pigeon Pose. In Sanskrit this is simply *Kapotasana*. Don't worry, we aren't going to perform this difficult and demanding backbend here. Instead, this Pigeon Pose variation is a restorative version most often used to open the hips. As such I've called this pose *Nidra Kapotasana*, Sleeping Pigeon Pose. The Sanskrit etymology can be a little confusing here so I wanted to be sure that you had the full story behind the pose.

Start off in Downward-Facing Dog. Keep your pelvic floor active and your lower abdominal muscles drawn in toward your spine. Inhale as you glide your right knee forward and settle your knee down on the outer edge of your right wrist. Keep your right toes pointing toward your left foot. Sink your left knee to the ground and keep your left hip joint in parallel position. Sink the weight of your hips toward the ground. Guide your pubic bone behind your right foot. Keep your knee joint closed if you feel tighter or if you feel any pressure around the knee. If your hips are comfortably settled on the ground and there is no discomfort in your knee joints, then you might be able to open your knee and place your shinbone parallel with the front of your yoga mat. This movement encourages a deeper external rotation of your right hip joint. But if your right hip joint is not yet open enough to facilitate this action, there may be some undue pressure on your knee. Be careful not to try and stretch your knee. In Pigeon Pose you are meant to target and stretch the muscles that control the movement of your hip joint. Deciding which placement of the shinbone is appropriate for your body, walk your hands forward and allow your chest and head to drape down toward the ground. Close your eyes and breathe deeply. Be very aware of all the sensations through your body. Stay for ten to fifty breaths. Return to Downward-Facing Dog and repeat on the other side.

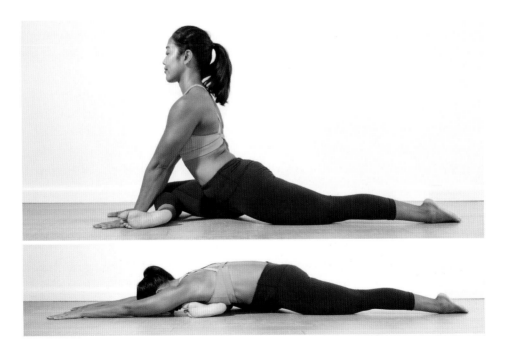

Pigeon on a Perch

Sometimes it can be impossible to get into either variation of Pigeon Pose without pressure on your knee. To make Pigeon Pose more accessible, and to create more space, try elevating your hands on blocks. Bring your right knee forward and wide, placing your knee to the right side of your mat. Adjust your right knee so that your right shin is positioned toward the front edge of your mat. Your right knee doesn't have to be parallel to the front of the mat, so if this is unavailable to you, find a position where you feel engagement in your right hip. Tuck your left toes under and lift your leg away from the mat. Keep both of your legs active by flexing and spreading your right toes while keeping your left toes pointing toward the back edge of your mat. Now try placing a block underneath your right hip. From here you can keep your body upright on your fingertips or you can fold forward onto your forearms.

Try using a bolster to create another variation of Pigeon Pose. Start in Downward-Facing Dog in a lunge, and then step your right foot over the bolster. Lower your left knee down to the mat. Now, align the heel and toes of your right foot to the left side of the mat, allowing your hip to rest on the bolster.

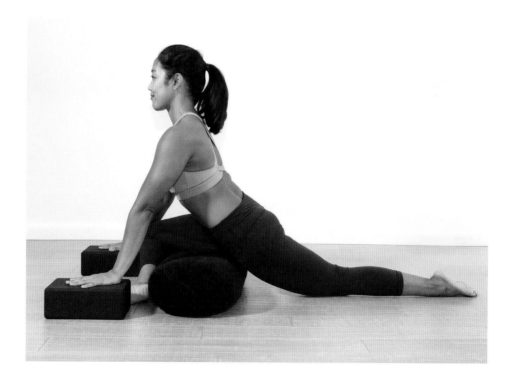

Pigeon on a Chair

If none of the options outlined above are accessible for you, there are still other ways for you to access this pose. Start off seated on a chair. Keep your pelvic floor engaged and your lower abdominal muscles drawn in. Draw your right knee into your chest and gently rest your right foot on the outer edge of your left lower thigh. Exhale as your right knee gently sinks and your right hip joint folds into external rotation. Fold your chest down toward your right shinbone. Stay for five breaths, then return to the seated position and repeat on the other side.

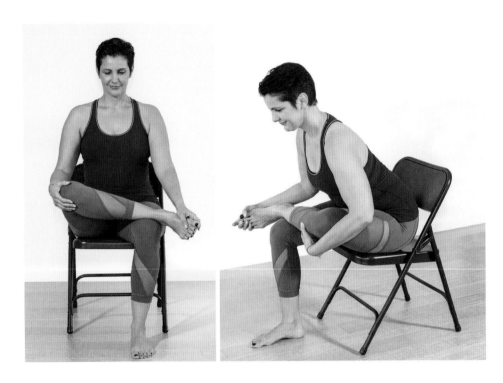

Side Plank Pose
Vashishtasana

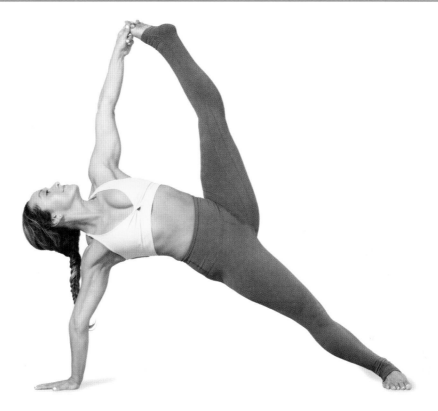

24

If you've taken a class with me, you know that I love Plank Pose! When in doubt I will always throw in a few planks. The reason that I love Plank Pose so much is that it's such an amazing tool to build strength. Side Plank Pose is a special plank because it is asymmetrical. Whenever you practice an asymmetrical pose, it is important to expect and accept differences in your body. No body is perfectly symmetrical, nor should it be. That being said, the best way to even out any structural differences in your body's strength is to practice asymmetrical strength poses for an equal length of time on both sides. There is no need to spend extra time on the side that is weaker. Over years of practice, both sides will find their natural equilibrium.

Side Plank Pose is based on the advanced yoga pose called *Vashishtasana*, the Pose Dedicated to the Sage Vashishta. There are many advanced variations of the Side Plank Pose, but I have chosen not to include them here in this pose progression. I find that students often skip the basics and aim for what appears to be advanced. It's a natural human tendency. To help you avoid the pitfalls that come from skipping over the foundational elements of strength and alignment in what develops into a very advanced pose, I ask you to stick to the basics here. In my personal practice I spend lots of time in the basics, building up Plank Pose and Side Plank Pose each day. While you may watch me practice online and see me execute some very skillful moves, the core of my practice is building up basic strength in easily accessible poses such as this one. There is no need to make the practice intimidating or overly advanced for it to be successful in effecting the awakening that is the heart of yoga.

◆◆◆◆◆◆ ◆ ◆◆◆◆◆◆

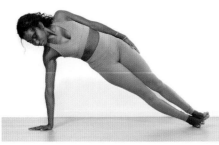

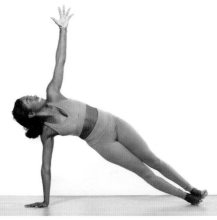

Start off in Plank Pose. Bring your feet together. Walk your right hand slightly forward, about a palm's length or less. Send your weight over to your right side and stack both feet on top of each other. Come on to your left fingertips and, once you feel stabile, lift your left hand off the ground and layer your arm along the left side of your body. Gaze down toward your right hand. Protract your right shoulder and push down into your right hand. Lift upward from deep within your torso, engaging your abdominal muscles with special attention on the internal obliques and the transverse abdominals.

Rotate your pelvis slightly under and hug your lower ribs in together. Avoid arching your back or bearing the load of your body in your back. Instead, use your core strength to draw the muscles of your body in toward the centerline, keep the foundation firm in your right arm and shoulder, and draw both legs together for increased stability. If you feel stable, then gently lift up your left arm.

Stack your shoulders in line with each other and reach up with your left fingertips. Gaze toward your left fingers. Stay for five breaths, then return to Plank Pose. Repeat on the other side.

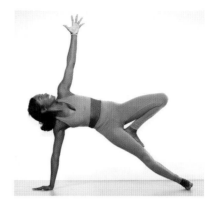

VARIATIONS
Side Plank with One Knee Down
Sometimes the shoulders aren't ready to carry the full weight of the body. If this is the case, take one knee down when rolling over to Side Plank. Following the instructions outlined above, place your right knee on the ground when rolling over to the right side. Slightly rotate your right hip joint to allow your right knee to find a stable base under your pelvis. While your right knee is used as support, avoid dumping weight down into your right knee. Instead, focus on pressing more strongly through your right shoulders and lifting up as much as possible.

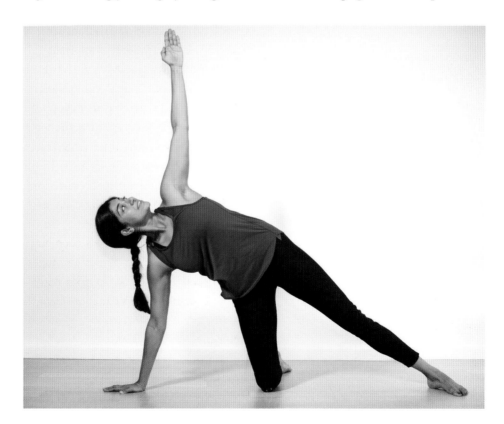

Forearm Side Plank

If you have a wrist injury or arthritis in your wrists, or if your shoulders are not very strong, Side Plank will be very challenging. Instead, try modifying Side Plank by using your forearms. The addition of the forearms makes for a more stable base. Start off on your hands and knees in modified Plank Pose. Place your elbows down, slightly less than shoulder-width apart. Step your feet back, activate your pelvic floor, and draw in your lower abdominal muscles. Inhale

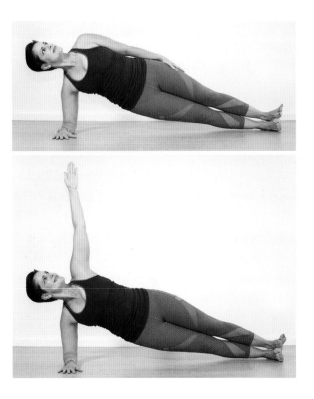

as you come up to the Forearm Plank Pose. Keep your back in a gentle spinal flexion. Rotate your right hand toward the left, bending at your elbow joint, and point your right fingers toward your left elbow. Draw in your lower ribs toward each other and inhale as you stack your body over to the right. Engage your core muscles with extra emphasis on serrates anterior, your transverse abdominals, and your internal obliques. Follow the same instructions outlined above for Side Plank.

Plow Pose

Halasana

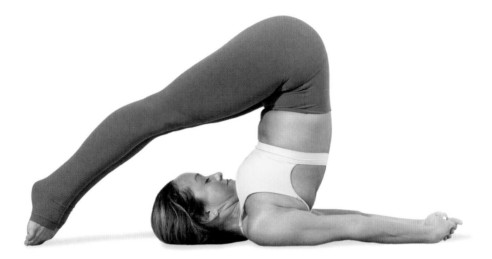

25

Inverting your body can be healing. It challenges you to think differently about your body. If you aren't used to being upside down, then even a little change of perspective may bring about a big change in your energy levels and sense of body awareness. Halasana, or Plow Pose, is one of the most accessible of the shoulder-stand group of poses. Regular practice of *Halasana* helps regulate the nervous system and stimulates the pituitary gland. While never a replacement for medical treatment, yoga poses have been shown to have therapeutic effect on the body and mind. Halasana is an introspective pose that encourages deep states of relaxation and stress relief.

◆ ◆ ◆ ◆ ◆ ◆ ◆ ◆ ◆ ◆ ◆ ◆ ◆

Lie flat on your back. Activate your pelvic floor and draw in your lower abdominal muscles toward your spine. Inhale as you gently lift your legs all the way over the top of your head. Roll your shoulders under so that the bulk of your trapezius and upper back presses in toward the ground. Extend your arms behind your back and interlace your fingers. Avoid flattening the back of your neck into the ground, but keep a bit of weight pressing down through the back of your head.

Align your hips with your shoulders and lift up along the central axis of your spine to keep your spine as straight as possible. Touch your toes down over the top of your head. Point your feet, straighten your legs, and firm your quadriceps. Fold forward by pivoting in through your hip joints. Rest your chin on your chest and gaze toward your nose. Stay for ten breaths, then release your hands, roll your spine down, and return to a full supine position.

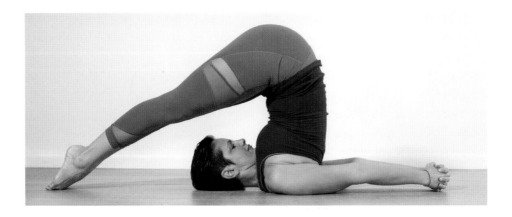

VARIATIONS
Plow Pose Using the Wall

To make Halasana more accessible, position yourself against a wall and use a folded blanket to support your shoulders. If you have a large chest, you may wish to secure your breasts with a strap. Lie flat on your back with your head facing toward the wall. Extend your legs and take your arms down along the sides of your torso. Press the palms of your hands down firmly into the floor as you engage your abdominal muscles. Inhale as you lift your legs and hips

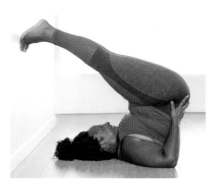

toward the ceiling. Place a block underneath your hips for added support. Straighten your legs and slowly lower your toes to the wall behind you. Tuck your shoulders underneath you and walk your feet lower down the wall. If your toes are close to touching the floor, try using blocks underneath your feet instead of using the wall. If you are not able to interlace your fingers behind your back, try holding on to a block or strap behind your back.

Plow Pose with Blanket Under Your Shoulders

Plow Pose and all the traditional shoulder-stand poses can be very challenging if you have a tight or sore neck. Other students may simply find that the back of the neck presses uncomfortably into the ground despite efforts to lift up and support the cervical spine. Using a blanket under your shoulders increases the amount of space between your shoulders and can relieve discomfort around your neck. Fold a blanket into a rectangle, making sure that the blanket is folded evenly. Place your shoulders on the long edge of the folded blanket and guide your shoulder blades under your back and onto the blanket. Allow your neck to hang off the blanket and gently touch the floor. Check the space between the cervical spine and the floor and adjust the height of the blanket, if necessary, to maximize this space. Use the blanket to form a stable base. Inhale as you activate the muscles of your pelvic floor, lift your body off the ground, draw your legs over the top of your head, point your toes as you lower them to the ground, interlock your fingers, and enter Halasana, Plow Pose.

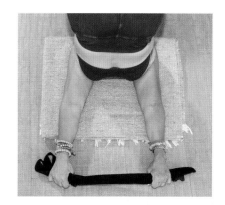

Plow Pose Using a Chair

If your feet do not touch the ground, you may find Halasana exceedingly uncomfortable and strenuous. Whether you lack the strength or flexibility, try using a chair to rest your feet on. Use a blanket if your neck needs the extra support or enter the pose without the additional support. To set up, place the chair behind where your head will be on the floor with the open front of the chair, where the seat is, facing forward toward your head. Following the same instructions listed above, enter Halasana, Plow Pose. Instead of reaching the feet to the ground, rest the tips of the toes on the chair. Since a relatively deep forward fold is required to allow your feet to touch the floor, elevating the contact point with the use of a chair lessens the burden of how deeply you need to fold.

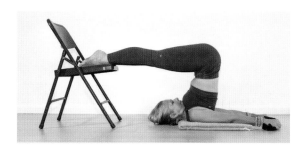

Since your feet are resting on a chair, there is also less pressure on your neck and shoulders. Similarly, since your feet do not touch the floor, less strength is needed to enter this variation. Using the chair for support may allow you to hold the pose for a slightly longer time and feel more at ease as you practice.

ALTERNATIVE TO PLOW POSE

Inverted Pose / Viparita Karani

If you have any neck issues, you are not advised to roll through your cervical spine. In this case, practice Viparita Karani, Inverted Pose, most often referred

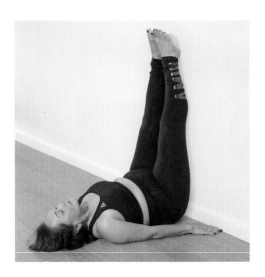

to simply as Legs Up Pose, as an alternative. Start off in a reclining position. Activate your pelvic floor and draw in your lower abdominal muscles toward your spine. Inhale as you gently lift your legs. Stack your legs in line with your hip joints and press the bases of your big toes together. Point your feet and spiral your thighs toward each other to encourage a gently internal rotation of your hip joints. Relax your neck and shoulders. Gaze toward your nose.

Headstand

Sirsasana

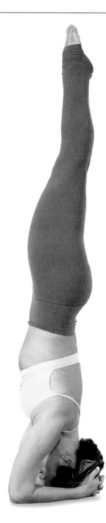

26

There is no point in stressing over things you can't control. The more you obsess about things that are outside of the realm of your power, the more anxious and out of control you feel. It can be hard in the midst of struggle to have faith in the bigger picture and trust that the universe really is working for the greater good and your good too. But that's exactly when all your training as a yogi matters most.

It took me nearly a year of practice before *Sirsasana*, or Headstand, started to happen regularly. There were days that it felt hopeless, and I stressed out about not being able to balance Headstand. I once tried this pose so many times that I lost count. It got worse and worse, and I was belligerent, punitive, and aggressive toward myself. One thing I learned along the way is that every pose has its time, just like every flower has its time. No amount of stressing, forcing, or pushing will change it. The key to a good practice is learning how to be at peace with yourself and your body right now, with whatever strength or lack thereof, whatever size or shape you are, and also to keep practicing with a heart full of love.

When things feel hopeless, when no path laid out before you leads to peace, when it all just feels difficult and exhausting, don't give up, but don't force it either. If you have done everything within your power and you still haven't reached your goal, the only thing left is to let it go. I can't tell you how hard this is for me. If I did, then so can you! It wasn't easy for me, so please don't get discouraged if you don't find your balance in Sirsasana after the first try or even after the first thousand tries. What matters is that you are working with intelligence and deep inner awareness. If there's a hint of shame and blame, it's probably a good indication that you're trying to force it. If you're feeling hopeful, joyful, expectant, energized, or peaceful, you are probably operating from love.

* * * * * * ◆ * * * * * *

Start off in Tabletop Pose. Activate your pelvic floor and draw in your lower abdominal muscles toward your spine. Drop your elbows to the ground, shoulder-width apart. Check your distance by hugging the outer edges of your opposite elbows with your fingertips. Interlace your fingers and open your palms. Firm your

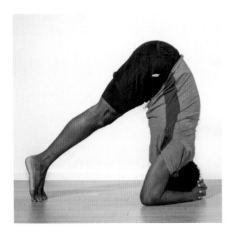

deltoids, root down into your elbows, and ground the outer edges of your palms. Place the top of your head on the floor and cradle the back of your head between your palms. Stabilizing your shoulder girdle, inhale as you straighten your legs. Gently walk your feet in toward your head. Stop when you reach a limit to your flexibility. Press even more into your elbows, draw your lower ribs in toward your spine, and engage all the muscles of your torso.

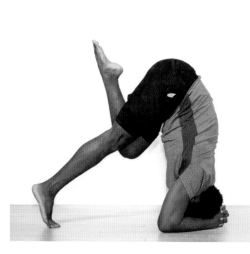
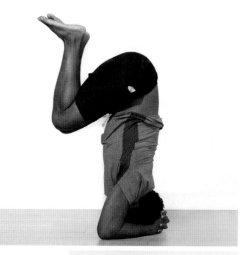

Inhale as you draw your left knee in toward your chest. Pivot your hips forward and slightly up. Feel the weight of your body transfer into the strength of your arms. This is called the "Prepare Pose" for the Headstand. Stay for a few breaths and switch sides. Inhale again as you lift or lightly jump your hips forward and up to bring both knees into your chest. Stay for a few breaths. If you remain in balance, extend your legs to enter Sirsasana. Stay for up to twenty-five breaths. Come down to Child's Pose. While the traditional gaze is toward the nose, I usually advise you to gaze outward to a single point while you are learning the basics of Headstand.

Don't feel any pressure to move immediately to Sirsasana. Instead, stay in the prepare for a long time to build strength.

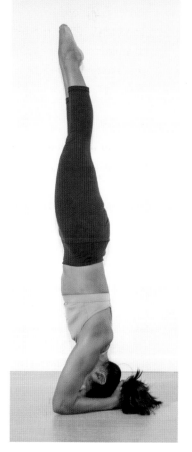

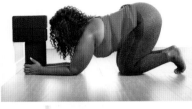

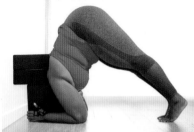

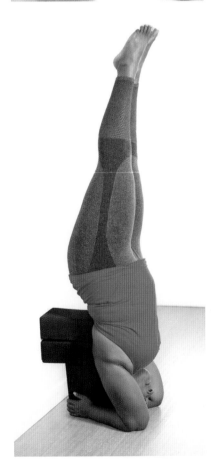

VARIATION
Headstand Hybrid

This variation of Headstand is a Forearm Headstand hybrid that is helpful for students who can't put weight on their heads. For this accessible Headstand variation, you will need three thick blocks and easy access to a sturdy wall. Place one block vertically, approximately one block length away from the wall, using the block's highest height setting. Then stack two blocks horizontally on top of the vertical block, placing the blocks flush with the wall.

Kneel on the floor in front of the blocks. Lace your fingers around the bottom block and set your forearms on the floor, placing your elbows directly under your shoulders. Set the back of your head against the blocks and push your forearms into the floor. Now walk your feet forward until your upper back is fully supported by all three blocks. Press down firmly with your forearms as you press your upper back into the blocks. Inhale and lift your feet away from the floor. Take both feet up at the same time, or lift one leg up at a time to find your balance. If there is no weight on your head, you can hop lightly off the floor while engaging your forearms and upper back. Squeeze your knees together and press down through your forearms.

Dolphin Pose / Zizumarasana

If you have glaucoma or a neck injury and are not placing weight on the top of your head, Dolphin Pose is a strength-building alternative that will give you similar benefits as Headstand. It's also great prep for Sirsasana.

Start off in Tabletop Pose. Activate your pelvic floor and draw in your lower abdominal muscles toward your spine. Drop your elbows to the ground, shoulder-width apart. Check your distance by hugging the outer edges of your opposite elbows with your fingertips. Stack your shoulders directly above your elbows. Press your forearms down firmly into the mat with your hands clasped together. Now tuck your toes under and come into Dolphin Pose. Keep your shoulders stacked directly above your elbows. Walk your feet forward toward your elbows. Gaze back toward your legs. Press down fully into your forearms and hug your outer forearms in toward each other. If you are fully engaged in your shoulders, your head will remain off the floor.

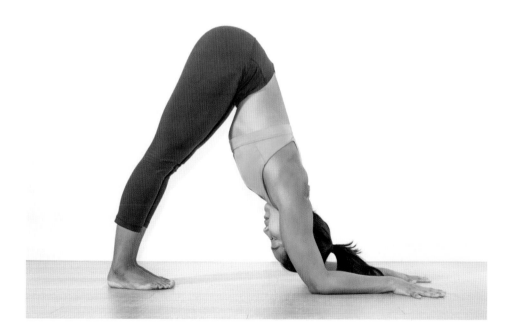

Warrior II
Virabhadrasana B

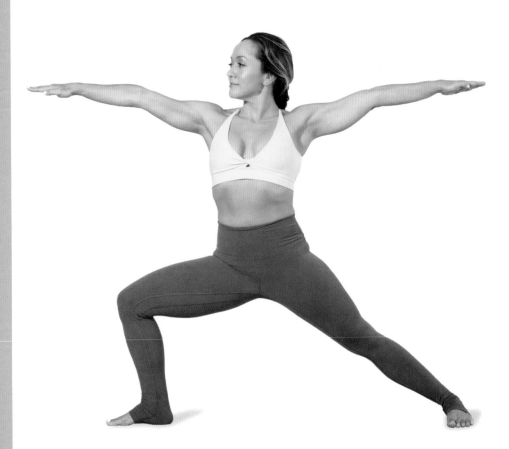

27

There are many ways to enter Virabhadrasana B, or Warrior II, depending on which type of practice you learn. In the Ashtanga yoga method, Virabhadrasana B is typically entered directly from Virabhadrasana A, or Warrior I. However, for ease of practice I will guide you through the instructions directly from Samasthiti. Feel welcome to string these two poses together in a flow once you're familiar with them both. Spending a little extra time building up the foundation and alignment in Virabhadrasana B helps strengthen the legs and builds endurance.

Start in Samasthiti. Activate your pelvic floor and draw in your lower abdominal muscles toward your spine. Inhale as you step out to the right, taking your feet between three and four feet apart. Start with your feet and hip joints parallel. Externally rotate your right hip joint and turn your right toes out to the side. Align your right heel with your left arch or your right heel with your left heel, whichever feels more stable. Keep your left toes pointed forward or even slightly toward the right. Bend your right knee over your right ankle and track your right knee, right hip, and right foot all in the same line. Even as your right knee bends, gently draw your right femur into its socket to encourage a slight hip flexion. Eventually your right thigh will be parallel with the ground, but please do not start there. Check your distance and always be sure that your hips do not drop below your bent knee and that your knee never extends beyond your toes in this pose. Root down firmly into both legs. Drop your hips and keep your tailbone heavy (but not tucked). Level your sitting bones and check to be sure that one hip is not higher than the other.

Abduct and lengthen your right inner thigh. Stack your rib cage over your hips and bring awareness to the centerline of your body. Send the center of your chest slightly up, broaden your collarbone, and extend your arms. Spread your shoulder blades away from each other, straighten your arms, and close your right fingers. Reach your arms away from each other and gaze toward your right fingers. Avoid leaning forward with your torso. Free your neck and keep lifting up along your spinal axis to maximize space between the joints of your spine. Stay for five breaths, then immediately pivot over to the left side. Stay for five breaths, then return to Samasthiti.

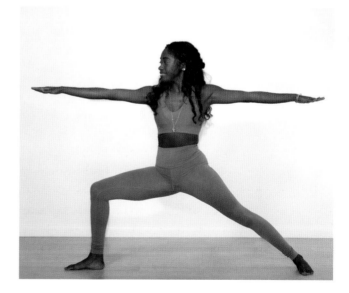

Warrior II with a Chair

Start off seated on a chair with both feet firmly planted on the ground and the hips shifted toward the very front of the chair. Be sure to use a chair that is the appropriate height so that your feet are not floating. Activate the muscles of the pelvic floor and be conscious of the placement of your hips. Extend the right leg outward and roll the right thigh bone back and down. Firmly press into the right foot and allow the chair to carry the weight of the body. Extend the left leg outward until the left foot is firmly planted on the ground and the left leg is straight. There will be a natural weight shift in the hips. Once you feel stable and supported by the chair, align the hips so that the sitting bones are on the same plane and one hip is not hiked above the other. After the legs and pelvis are settled, lift the spine upward along its axis to maximize the space between the ribs and the hips. Extend the arms outward, parallel with the ground to a T shape. Gaze toward the right hand. Stay for five breaths, then switch the sides.

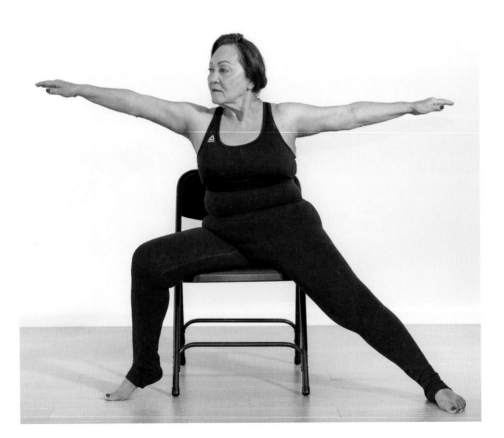

Warrior II on the Wall

Sometimes both balance and body awareness may be difficult. If you find it hard to feel your body, try using the wall to enter Virabhadrasana B. Start in Samasthiti with your back facing the wall. Move as close to the wall as feels comfortable. Follow the instructions outlined above, setting your hips and possibly also your torso onto the wall for additional support.

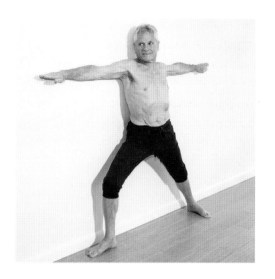

Warrior II with Hands on Your Waist

If your shoulders are injured, it may be difficult to raise your arms. Similarly, if you find it challenging to feel your hips, it may be useful to use your arms as anchors to support the alignment of your pelvis. Follow the instructions outlined above, then, instead of raising your arms, take your hands to your hips. Use your hands to guide your hips into alignment. If your hips settle, try bringing your hands to prayer position at the center of your chest. Gaze toward your nose. Stay for five breaths and repeat on the other side.

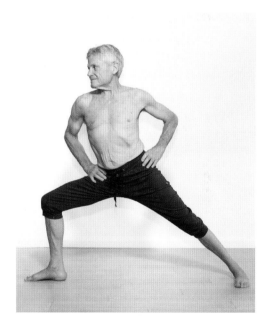

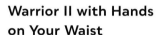

Warrior II Not Down as Far

Sometimes bending the knees too deeply may be difficult for arthritic or otherwise sensitive knees. Similarly, going down too far into the legs may be challenging for those with bad balance or less strength in the legs. An easy alternative is to simply not go down as far into Warrior II. Enter the pose following the same instructions outlined above except set up with a slightly narrower stance and do not bend the forward leg as much as indicated above. Instead, find a comfortable spot that allows you to work with intelligence and ease.

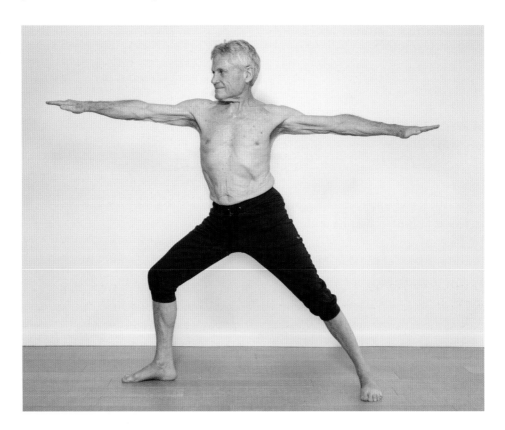

Pendant Pose

Lolasana

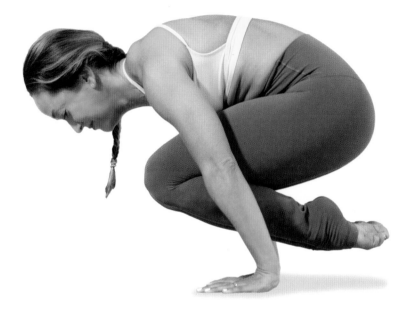

28

Lolasana, or Pendant Pose, is a difficult asana that requires full engagement of your entire body. Your abdominal muscles, back muscles, and shoulders are all part of the equation here. I personally struggle with Lolasana and understand how frustrating it feels to push into the ground with all your strength and have no lift-up happen. If you're like me, you will need to find creative ways to practice Lolasana as you build strength. But one thing is certain, if I could build the strength, then so can you! I wasn't naturally strong when I started the practice. I was never a gymnast or a dancer; all the strength I have today is from years of practice.

So many students think that they need superlong arms in order to find the lift-up in Lolasana. While long arms may give you an advantage, they aren't the deciding factor. I, for one, do not have particularly long arms and I eventually found the strength to lift up in Lolasana. There is perhaps no greater core strength challenge than this! Let the journey of strength be far more than physical. Dive deeply within yourself and let the journey of strength transform your soul.

Start off in Child's Pose. Gently lift your torso but leave your body seated on your feet. Place your hands flat on the floor behind your knees. Activate your pelvic floor and engage your abdominal muscles. Spread your shoulder blades away from each other and straighten your arms. Round your back and hug in your lower ribs toward the centerline. Push down through your arms and engage the same muscular activation as in Plank Pose. Inhale as you adduct your thighs and draw in your knees toward your chest. Keep both feet on the ground. Gaze forward and slightly down. Push from your shoulders, send your chest slightly forward, and lift

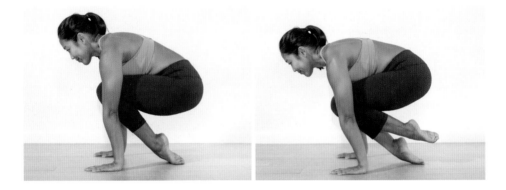

one foot off the ground. Stay for a few breaths, then switch feet. Finally, send your shoulders and chest forward, engage your core muscles even stronger, and adduct your thighs to lift both feet off the ground. Think about working the opposing forces of sending your shoulders forward and down while lifting your hips back and slightly up. Gaze forward. Stay for five breaths. Come down and repeat two more times.

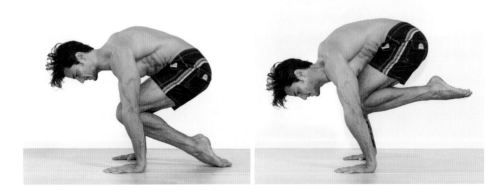

Pendant Pose with Blocks

To make Lolasana more accessible, use a block under each hand. Choose the height for the blocks that allows your arms to remain long but not hyperextended. If you don't have two blocks, try using two chairs that are the same height. Follow the same instructions outlined above.

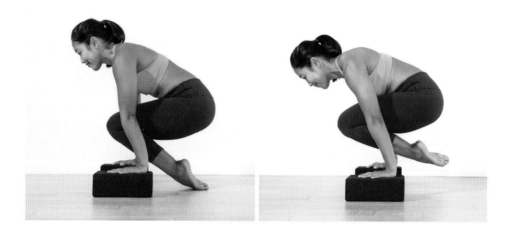

Reclining Twist

Supta Ardha Matsyendrasana

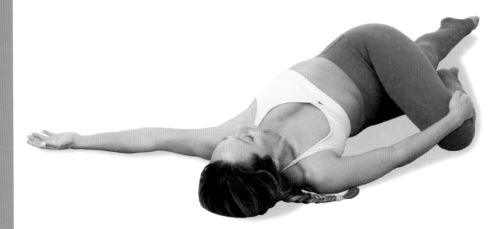

29

Some of the deepest experiences during your yoga practice may not happen in dynamic poses. The meditative state of mind achieved while staying for long holds in more restorative poses allows the body and mind to rest in unity. Completing your journey with a softer approach to the practice helps your mind make the transition to meditation and contemplation. I encourage you to always practice a combination of strong and soft poses, balancing the yin and the yang in each practice. Traditionally, Patanjali advises yoga students to find the balance between practice (*abhyasa*) and surrender (*vairagya*). By taking a dynamic twisting pose into a relaxed stance, it allows you to access a deeper dimension of your meditative mind during the practice. Reclining Twist is a deconstructed version of the more dynamic twisting pose called *Ardha Matsyendrasana*, Half Lord of the Fishes Pose. In Reclining Twist pose, place your emphasis on surrender and release all resistance. Enter your inner body by keeping your mind focused on the subtle sensations that arise without any judgment.

◆◆◆◆◆◆ ◆ ◆◆◆◆◆◆

Lie on your back, arms along your sides. Activate your pelvic floor and draw in your lower abdominal muscles toward your spine. Inhale as you draw your right knee in toward your chest. Stabilize your left leg and root down with your left heel. Wrap your left hand around your right shin, just under your knee. Lift your ribs away from your hips while keeping your pelvis grounded. Exhale as you gently twist your body to the left, initiating the motion by bringing your right knee across your body's centerline. Extend your right arm to counterbalance your weight. Gaze to the right. Do not force your right knee or right hand to the ground. Simply allow your body to find a comfortable position to release and rest. Keep your left leg active and reaching away. Stay for five to twenty breaths and then switch sides.

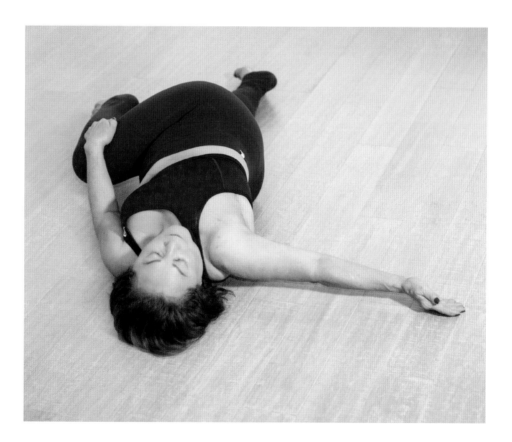

Reclining Twist with Support

If your head, neck, knee, and arm experience severe discomfort, it is not recommended to suffer so intensively. Instead, support your bent knee and extended arm by placing a block, bolster, or pillow under them.

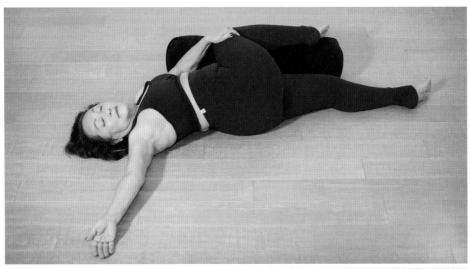

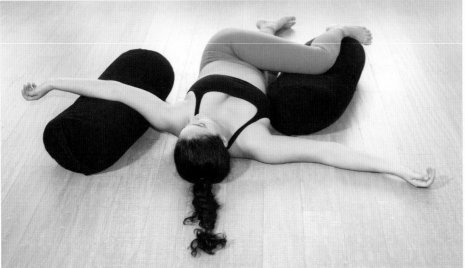

Meditation Pose

Sukhasana

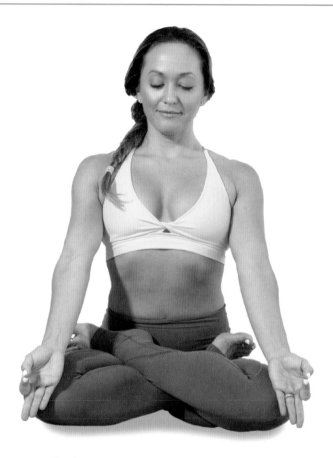

30

Sukhasana, or Meditation Pose, can be done in any seated position, whether on the floor or in a chair. The most important thing is to find a seated position that is comfortable. If you begin with discomfort, it will be impossible to hold the same position for an extended period of time. I like to end each practice with a few moments of contemplative introspection to help integrate the deep spiritual learning that happens within each practice.

◆ ◆ ◆ ◆ ◆ ◆ ◆ ◆ ◆ ◆ ◆ ◆ ◆

Start off in Dandasana. Activate your pelvic floor and draw in your lower abdominal muscles toward your spine. Bend your knees out to the sides and externally rotate your hip joints. Place your feet on the floor one in front of the other. Avoid stacking the feet on top of each other, folding the ankles onto the thighs, or any other position that places pressure on your feet or ankles. Since we aim to hold Meditation Pose for around five minutes without moving, it is best to start off with as little discomfort in or stress on any of the joints in your body. Place your

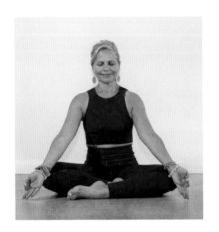

hands on your knees. Pivot slightly forward into your hip joints. Allow your rib cage to gently float away from your hips and send your chest slightly forward. Avoid looking up or letting your head hang on your shoulders like a hinge. Instead, let your head be supported by positioning it well above your spine. Keep your collarbone broad. While finding a comfortable position is best when the anatomical arrangement of your body is aligned, entering a meditative state also includes a sense of detachment to your physical form. So, do your best, but don't obsess about the details.

VARIATIONS
Meditation Pose with Support
Take any crossed-legged seated position that you can commit to for a set length of time. Use cushions, blocks, or blankets to lift your hips and support your knees.

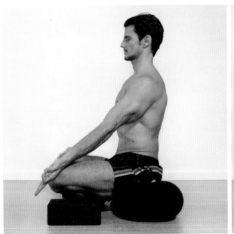
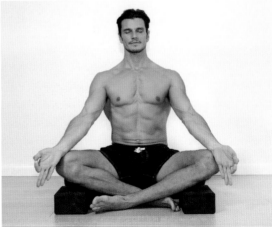

Find a position in which you feel comfortable. Elongate your spine. An elevated seat will help keep your back straight and avoid pinching your neck and shoulders. When your seat is elevated, only your feet will rest on the floor. Allow your hips to soften and your knees to descend toward the floor. You may find that you only need to elevate your hips in order to find comfort. Or you may find that you only need to support your knees to find comfort. Experiment with the option that is right for your body. Relax your shoulders and jaw. Follow the instructions outlined above.

Meditation Pose on a Chair

Sit in a chair or stool where your feet reach comfortably to the ground. Shift slightly forward on the seat so that your back is not supported by the backrest. Allow the natural curvature of your spine to be expressed. Avoid slouching or scrunching your shoulders and neck. Follow the instructions outlined above.

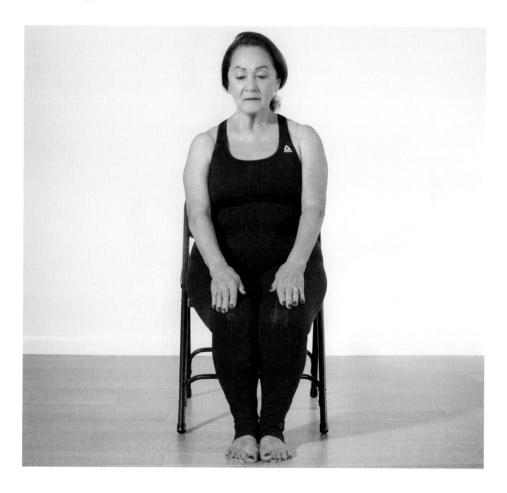

Constructive Rest Pose

Vizramasana

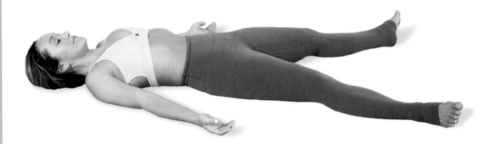

Constructive Rest Pose is a very important practice. It helps us get centered and allows asana practice to do its work. At the end of a challenging practice, my teachers in India used to say that it was now time to "take rest." *Vizramasana* literally means "Take Rest Pose" and refers to the final relaxation pose in your practice. Outside of the Ashtanga yoga tradition, this pose is often referred to as *Savasana*. Popularized by the Alexander Technique Method, Constructive Rest allows the spine, back muscles, and nervous system to truly rest and recuperate. Use two blocks, a bolster, and a blanket to create a Constructive Rest Pose that is accessible and relaxing.

* * * * * * ◆ * * * * * *

Place the blocks underneath the bolster, with one block on its highest height setting so that it gives you as much height as possible. For added support, rest the second block on its long side, placing the block in the middle of the bolster. Carefully lean your back onto the elevated bolster. For extra support, you can place a cushion or a rolled blanket underneath your neck or at your lower back.

Experiment with arm and hand placements as well as support under your knees. You can also bring the soles of your feet together in Butterfly Pose. There are lots of ways to take Constructive Rest Pose. Try lying in Vizramasana with a bolster under your knees and a cushion under your neck. Find a place where you can be comfortable and enjoy the rest.

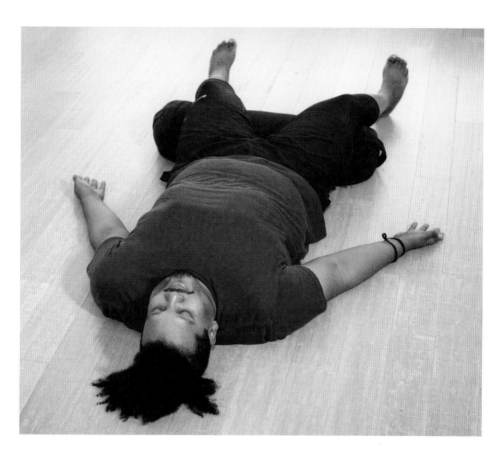

For the bottom half of your body, you could take Baddha Konasana legs (Butterfly Pose), or extend the legs in Vizramasana.

143

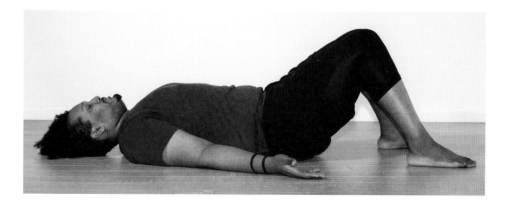

student bios

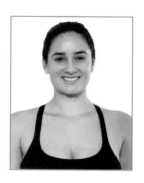

MONICA ARELLANO

Monica Arellano first connected with the practice of yoga in 2010. She graduated from Miami Life Center's Ashtanga Practitioner's Intensive Course in 2016 and MLC's apprenticeship program in 2018, both under the guidance of Tim Feldmann and Kino MacGregor. She makes the journey to Mysore, India, annually to study at the source with R. Sharath Jois. Today she is a student, teacher, and manager at Miami Life Center.

Coming to the mat six times a week, Monica allows the experience of the practice to guide her, alongside the knowledge carried on from her teachers. Through an asana and meditation practice, she explores the movement of the breath and a calm and sharp mind, continuously seeking a balance between effort and surrender. For Monica, yoga is the lifelong cultivation and integration of these skills in body, mind, and spirit.

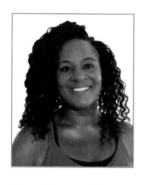

DIANNE BONDY

Dianne Bondy is a celebrated yoga teacher, social justice activist, and leading voice of the Yoga For All movement. Her inclusive view of yoga asana and philosophy inspires and empowers thousands of followers around the world—regardless of their shape, size, ethnicity, or level of ability. Dianne contributes to Yoga International, Do You Yoga, and Elephant Journal. She is featured and profiled in international media outlets including the *Guardian*, *Huffington Post*, *Cosmopolitan*, *People*, and more. She is a spokesperson for diversity in yoga and yoga for larger bodies, as seen in her work with Pennington's, Gaiam, and the Yoga & Body Image Coalition. Her work is published in the books *Yoga and Body Image*, *Yes Yoga Has Curves*, and *Yoga Where You Are*.

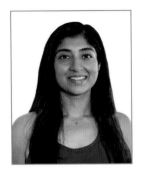

SAIRA FIDA

Born and raised in Clearwater, Florida, Saira is an Indian American who enjoys Florida's natural beauty and seeks to protect it. Saira is a cofounder and treasurer of Debris Free Oceans (DFO), a Miami-based 501(c)(3) nonprofit dedicated to inspiring local communities to reduce their daily waste stream (www.debrisfreeoceans.org). She dreams of Miami becoming a zero-waste community. Saira incorporates sustainability into her daily life and appreciates communities that come together to bring systemic change and transition from convenience living to making sustainable choices seamless and effortless. Saira finds yoga brings the stillness to her life that she is desperately seeking. After many years of practicing, she continues to find the simplest yoga asana challenging. Each time she comes to her mat, she finds she opens her "inflexible" body a little bit more, finding that a tiny bit more space is available. Saira hopes those who feel yoga is only for the most fit and flexible will now consider committing to giving it a try. Over time, with consistency of practice and patience, yoga just might become the magic moment to add to your daily routine that you never knew you needed and can no longer live without.

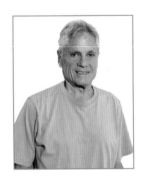

MARK LINKSMAN

Mark has had a lifelong passion for pursuing physical disciplines, specifically in body-mind systems. He combines playfulness with a deep understanding of the body. With twenty-five years of Shotokan Karate, then a student of BKS Iyengar in Pune/India, more than twenty years of Ashtanga yoga practice under Richard Freeman and Tim Miller, along with a daily self practice of asana, pranayama, and meditation, Mark has a lifetime of deeply ingrained wisdom in both body and mind. A special love for the breath has kept Mark's practice of pranayama close to his heart all days, a love first kindled by his teacher Tim Miller. Mark has taught a variety of asana and pranayama classes around the United States, but specifically at Tim Miller's Ashtanga Yoga Center in Encinitas and at the Miami Life Center.

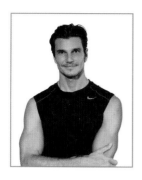

AITOR MATEO

Aitor is a Latin model, based in Miami, who is just starting his yoga journey.

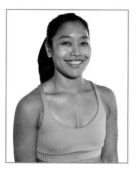

CHALISA NA NAKORNPANOM

When I first practiced yoga, I didn't know what I wanted to do was part of yoga. I wanted to do a handstand, and this opened the door to where I finally am now, an Ashtanga yoga practitioner.

I started off with a home practice by myself, then came across yoga challenges on Instagram, which led me to the Ashtanga method.

I'm from Thailand. I practice because it's what I love, and it's already part of my life—even if sometimes I don't feel like doing it. The practice is like water to me. Sometimes I feel so thirsty, and the water tastes so delicious. But other times it doesn't taste good, and I still have to drink it because my body needs it—and at the end of the day, I never regret drinking water! Just like I never regret practicing yoga.

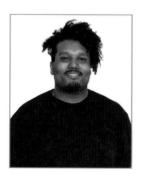

JAIME SKYE ORTEGA

Born February 9, 1992, in South Beach, Miami, Jaime grew up as a very observant individual. He learned life skills from those closest to him, including cooking from his mother, drawing from his older brother, and physical activities from his father. His family took note of their child's ability and passion for the arts and cultivated it. He went on to attend dedicated art classes and art schools. Jaime moved to New York to attend Parsons, the New School, and he graduated with a bachelor of fine arts degree. He entered the fashion world and designs gowns, swimwear, outerwear, and other collections, as well as creates portraits of people and pets. Jaime was encouraged to take a yoga class by his older brother two years ago and has been practicing four to five days a week ever since.

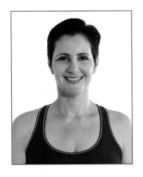

LINDA PEDROSO

Linda is fascinated with the human body and mind. She has dedicated her life to being a student and guide using yoga as her main tool. She believes that yoga can be used to heal the body-mind apparatus. It is a portal to meet the true self.

Her fitness career has spanned over a decade and included many modalities including but not limited to Pilates, personal training, spinning, and CrossFit. All of these modalities inform her practice and teaching. She has traveled with Grammy award–winning artists as a personal health coach and completed several international concert tours. She believes in the power of yoga and meditation to keep us grounded and centered.

Linda has a 200-hour training from 305Yoga in Miami under Terri Cooper and Claire Santos. She received her 300-hour from Anand Mehrotra in Rishikesh, India, at Sattva Yoga Academy.

She has also traveled extensively to ensure she always remains a student under the best teachers in the world. Her yogic studies have granted her the opportunity to practice with Sharath Jois, Dharma Mittra, Seane Corn, Shiva Rea, Schuyler Grant, Richard Freeman, Manju Jois, Marie Belle Perez Rivero, and David Swenson.

A Cuban American, she now resides once again in her hometown of Miami. It is truly a gift to be home and have the boon to be a student at Miami Life Center. She practices Ashtanga Mysore with Tim Feldman and Emilia Arenas.

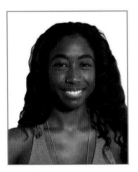

ELIZABETH RICHARDSON

Elizabeth is a retired dancer, active meditator, and passionate yogi. She's also a talented musician and an inspiration for following one's heart to achieve any goal or dream! Her journey into wellness didn't come easy—as they rarely do. She recalls a period during her college years where she was overworked, overwhelmed with stress, and unable to sleep—so much so, in fact, that she found she was often unfocused, disoriented, and living the life of an insomniac. Turning to meditation, a practice she learned early in life, she began to find relief. Combined with practicing pranayama and silencing her mind each night, it was as if everything began to fall into place. Along with igniting her breath, she found the moving meditation of Vinyasa-style yoga to be the missing piece that connected her history of movement and music together. Like dance, it gave her an outlet to express her creativity and release any tensions while increasing her energy and sense of well-being. Combining her love and talent for music, movement, and meditation, she was able to find herself again. She encourages her students to "let their breath be their music, and the music lead their movement." This mantra was her guide to self-discovery, and one she openly shares with all. After three years of a dedicated practice, she watched her quality of life improve. Her fears and insecurities began to fade. She was, in her words, simply happier! Taking her passion for yoga forward, she earned a 200-hour certification in Vinyasa power yoga. Along with teaching at SOL Yoga, she plans to further her practice and studies introducing yoga in new ways to the community, through inspiring music and powerful movement.

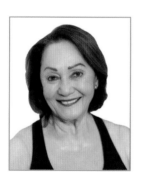

KINO MARY SAKUMA-MACGREGOR

Kino Sakuma-MacGregor is a Japanese American, born in 1943 in New York City. She was raised by her Japanese father, Suki, who moved their small family to Florida in the 1950s. Her early career as an activist and organizer for the Teachers' Union resulted in the passage of the collective bargaining law in Florida and granted early retirement benefits to teachers, among many other benefits. When her campaign to speak truth to power against the corruption of the leadership fell on deaf ears, she left the Teacher's Union. Working at Prudential, Sakuma-MacGregor hit another glass ceiling when, despite being the top performer in sales, she was not promoted. Deciding to finally become her own boss, she bought All American Insurance Associates, Inc., where she oversees a dedicated team that sells property and casualty insurance and excels in customer service and personalized client care. Sakuma-MacGregor was married to John Richard MacGregor for fifty-three years until he passed away. They shared a life of love, travel, orchids, rescue dogs, and, of course, their daughter, Kino MacGregor. After two total knee replacements, at the age of 75, she took her first yoga class and is currently working on Sun Salutation A and B.

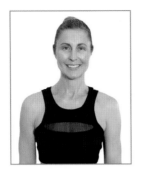

EDITA TOSMUK

I moved to Miami from Russia in 2007. Two years later, I started practicing Ashtanga yoga at the Miami Life Center. After several years of practice, I began to understand that yoga is a healing discipline for my mind and body, and realized that yoga changed my life in so many different ways. After eight years of practice, I decided that I could start sharing my experience of Ashtanga yoga with others. I started an apprenticeship in MCL's two-year training program, and by the end of the training in August 2017, I received the 200-hour yoga teacher certification. My goal is to become the type of teacher that will be able to identify the strengths as well as the challenges of each practitioner and guide them to achieve their personal goals, well-being, and healing.

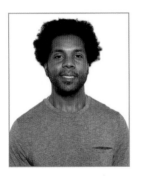

PATRICK R. TRACEY

Born March 27, 1985, in Port Antonio, Jamaica, Tracey immigrated to Miami Beach at an early age and considers himself "Miami grown." Tracey values learning and connection as well as making an impact in all he does. Travel is a passion for him that leads to new experiences in culture, ideas, and food. Music is a form of emotional expression and, as a DJ, he connects with others in an open-format style, mixing different genres to present his unique music. Tracey primarily works as a project manager in up-and-coming technology companies, including prattis.com, a subscription website aimed at management and agency development. Tracey loves sports and is a big Manchester United fan. He has had a passion for yoga for over five years now and loves to spread the benefits of yoga for mental and physical balance to all.

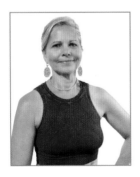

LISA FAREMOUTH WEBER

Lisa Faremouth Weber, E-RYT, RCYP is a certified yoga teacher and teacher trainer for both adults and children. Lisa also recently completed Level II Shiatsu Massage training. She opened Heaven Meets Earth Yoga Studio in 2005 located on Central Street in Evanston, Illinois. Lisa has developed her intuitive healing ability and shares that awareness through her yoga classes, private sessions, and consultations. She has studied with the top yoga instructors in the country including Rodney Yee, David Life, Baron Baptiste, Beryl Bender Birch, David Swenson, John Friend, Erich Shiffman, Stephen Cope, Bryan Kest, Shiva Rhea, Duncan Wong, Shakta Kaur Khalsa, Gurhmuhk and more. Lisa graduated from Northwestern University and completed her yoga instructor training at Moksha Yoga in Chicago. Prior to teaching yoga, Lisa was a certified personal trainer and group exercise leader traveling worldwide leading fitness training workshops. She is a published author and media producer. Lisa received her spiritual name, Sat Inder Kaur from Yogi Bhajan in 2004.

list of poses

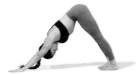

1. Downward-Facing Dog

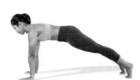

2. Plank Pose

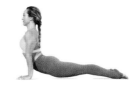

3. Upward-Facing Dog

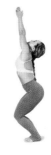

4. Chair Pose

5. Wide-Legged Forward Fold

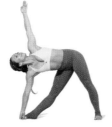

6. Triangle Pose

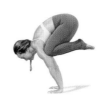

7. Crane Pose

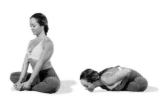

8. Butterfly Pose

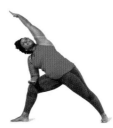

9. Extended Side Angle Pose

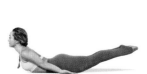

10. Locust Pose

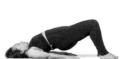

11. Simple Bridge Pose

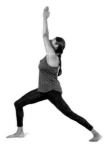

12. Warrior I

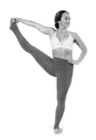

13. Standing Hand-to-Big-Toe Pose

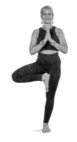

14. Tree Pose

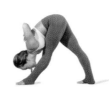

15. Pyramid Pose

16. Seated Forward Fold

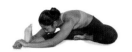

17. Head-to-Knee Pose

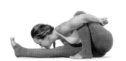

18. Marichi's Pose A

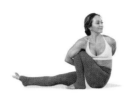

19. Marichi's Pose C

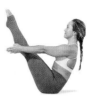

20. Boat Pose

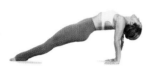

21. Reverse Plank

22. Camel Pose

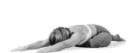

23. Pigeon Pose

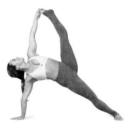

24. Side Plank Pose

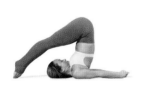

25. Plow Pose

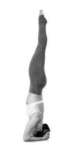

26. Headstand

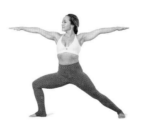

27. Warrior II

28. Pendant Pose

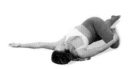

29. Reclining Twist

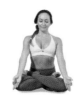

30. Meditation Pose

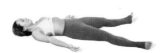

Bonus Pose
Constructive Rest Pose

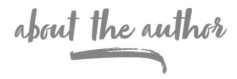

about the author

KINO MACGREGOR is a Miami native who is happiest on the beach with a fresh coconut. A poet at heart who always stops to smell the flowers, she is the founder of Omstars—the world's first yoga TV network, where you can practice with Kino live (www.omstars.com). With over 1 million followers on Instagram and over 600,000 subscribers on YouTube and Facebook, Kino's message of spiritual strength reaches people all over the world. Sought after as an expert in yoga worldwide, she is an international yoga teacher, inspirational speaker, author of four books, producer of six Ashtanga yoga DVDs, writer, world traveler, and cofounder of Miami Life Center.

Yoga for Kino is more than just a "workout"—it is a way life founded on a firm commitment to the moral and ethical precepts of truth, nonviolence, and love. For Kino, being strong in yoga is not just about a powerful handstand or a deep backbend, nor is yoga a game of extreme ableism where yogis compete with one another. Instead, Kino sees yoga as a daily ritual where people tune deeply into their spiritual center and experience the peace of the Eternal Divine. Kino believes in making the tools of traditional yoga accessible for all different sizes, shapes, ethnicities and ages and writes a popular blog that takes the lessons learned off the mat into real life. Rather than it being an exclusive club for the privileged elite, yoga is for everyone. It is the international community of yogis who are responsible for the integrity of the sacred heart of yoga.